Autoimmune Diseases of the Skin

Guest Editor

DÉDÉE F. MURRELL, MA, BMBCh, FAAD, MD, FACD

IMMUNOLOGY AND ALLERGY CLINICS OF NORTH AMERICA

www.immunology.theclinics.com

Consulting Editor
RAFEUL ALAM, MD, PhD

May 2012 • Volume 32 • Number 2

SAUNDERS an imprint of ELSEVIER, Inc.

W.B. SAUNDERS COMPANY

A Division of Elsevier Inc.

1600 John F. Kennedy Blvd., ● Suite 1800 ● Philadelphia, PA 19103-2899.

http://www.theclinics.com

IMMUNOLOGY AND ALLERGY CLINICS OF NORTH AMERICA Volume 32, Number 2

May 2012 ISSN 0889–8561, ISBN-13: 978-1-4557-5063-4

Editor: Pamela Hetherington

Immunology and Allergy Clinics of North America (ISSN 0889–8561) is published quarterly by Elsevier Inc., 360 Park Avenue South, New York, NY 10010-1710. Months of issue are February, May, August, and November. Periodicals postage paid at New York, NY and additional mailing offices. Subscription prices are $294.00 per year for US individuals, $417.00 per year for US institutions, $139.00 per year for US students and residents, $361.00 per year for Canadian individuals, $202.00 per year for Canadian students, $518.00 per year for Canadian institutions, $409.00 per year for international individuals, $518.00 per year for international institutions, $202.00 per year for international students. To receive student/resident rate, orders must be accompanied by name of affiliated institution, date of term, and the *signature* of program/residency coordinator on institution letterhead. Orders will be billed at individual rate until proof of status is received. Foreign air speed delivery is included in all *Clinics* subscription prices. All prices are subject to change without notice. **POSTMASTER**: Send address changes to *Immunology and Allergy Clinics of North America,* Elsevier Health Sciences Division, Subscription Customer Service, 3251 Riverport Lane, Maryland Heights, MO 63043. **Customer Service: 1-800-654-2452 (U.S. and Canada); 314-447-8871 (outside U.S. and Canada). Fax: 314-447-8029. E-mail: journalscustomerservice-usa@elsevier.com (for print support); journalsonlinesupport-usa@elsevier.com (for online support).**

Reprints. For copies of 100 or more, of articles in this publication, please contact the Commercial Reprints Department, Elsevier Inc., 360 Park Avenue South, New York, New York 10010-1710. Tel. (212) 633-3812, Fax: (212) 462-1935, E-mail: reprints@elsevier.com.

Immunology and Allergy Clinics of North America is covered in MEDLINE/PubMed (Index Medicus), Current Contents/Life Sciences, Science Citation Index, ISI/BIOMED, Chemical Abstracts, and EMBASE/Excerpta Medica.

Printed and bound by CPI Group (UK) Ltd, Croydon, CR0 4YY

Transferred to Digital Print 2012

Contributors

CONSULTING EDITOR

RAFEUL ALAM, MD, PhD
Veda and Chauncey Ritter Chair in Immunology, Professor, and Director, Division of Immunology and Allergy, National Jewish Health; and University of Colorado Health Sciences Center, Denver, Colorado

GUEST EDITOR

DÉDÉE F. MURRELL, MA, BMBCh, FAAD, MD, FACD
Professor and Head of Dermatology, St George Hospital, University of New South Wales, Kogarah, Sydney, New South Wales, Australia

AUTHORS

STEFAN BEISSERT, MD
Department of Dermatology, University of Muenster, Muenster, Germany

LUCA BORRADORI, MD
Department of Dermatology, Inselspital, University Hospital of Bern, Bern, Switzerland

ADELA RAMBI G. CARDONES, MD
Assistant Professor, Department of Dermatology, Duke University Medical Center, Durham, North Carolina

SHIEN-NING CHEE, MBBS (UNSW)
Department of Dermatology, St George Hospital, Kogarah; Faculty of Medicine, University of New South Wales, Kensington, Sydney, New South Wales, Australia

BENJAMIN S. DANIEL, BA, BCom, MBBS, MMed (Clin Epi)
Dermatology Research Fellow, Department of Dermatology, St George Hospital, Kogarah; Conjoint Associate Lecturer, Faculty of Medicine, University of New South Wales, Sydney, New South Wales, Australia

MICHAEL DAVID, MD
Professor, Department of Dermatology, Rabin Medical Center, Petah Tikva; Department of Dermatology, Sackler Faculty of Medicine, Tel Aviv University, Tel Aviv, Israel

ROCCO DELLA TORRE, MD
Department of Dermatology, Inselspital, University Hospital of Bern, Bern, Switzerland

MARINA ESKIN-SCHWARTZ, MD, PhD
Resident, Department of Dermatology, Rabin Medical Center, Petah Tikva; Department of Dermatology, Sackler Faculty of Medicine, Tel Aviv University, Tel Aviv, Israel

JOHN W. FREW, MBBS, MMed (Clin Epi)
Resident Medical Officer, St George Hospital, Kogarah; Faculty of Medicine, University of Sydney, Sydney, New South Wales, Australia

RUSSELL P. HALL III, MD
J. Lamar Callaway Professor and Chair, Department of Dermatology, Duke University
Medical Center, Durham, North Carolina

PASCAL JOLY, MD, PhD
Professor, Dermatology Department, INSERM U905, Rouen University Hospital,
Rouen, France

SAROLTA KÁRPÁTI, MD, PhD, DrSc
Professor, Department of Dermatology, Venereology and Dermato-Oncology,
Semmelweis University; Hungarian Academy of Sciences, Molecular Research Group,
Budapest, Hungary

VOLKER MEYER, MD
Department of Dermatology, University of Muenster, Muenster, Germany

DANIEL MIMOUNI, MD
Professor, Department of Dermatology, Rabin Medical Center, Petah Tikva; Department
of Dermatology, Sackler Faculty of Medicine, Tel Aviv University, Tel Aviv, Israel

DÉDÉE F. MURRELL, MA, BMBCh, FAAD, MD, FACD
Professor and Head of Dermatology, St George Hospital, University of New South Wales,
Kogarah, Sydney, New South Wales, Australia

WATARU NISHIE, MD, PhD
Department of Dermatology, Hokkaido University Graduate School of Medicine, Kita-ku,
Sapporo, Japan

EVAN W. PIETTE, MD
Department of Dermatology, University of Pennsylvania, Philadelphia, Pennsylvania

ENNO SCHMIDT, MD, PhD
Department of Dermatology; Comprehensive Center for Inflammation Medicine,
University of Lübeck, Lübeck, Germany

HIROSHI SHIMIZU, MD, PhD
Department of Dermatology, Hokkaido University Graduate School of Medicine, Kita-ku,
Sapporo, Japan

HIDEYUKI UJIIE, MD, PhD
Department of Dermatology, Hokkaido University Graduate School of Medicine, Kita-ku,
Sapporo, Japan

VANESSA A. VENNING, BMBCh, DM, FRCP
Consultant Dermatologist and Honorary Senior Lecturer, Department of Dermatology,
Churchill Hospital, Oxford, United Kingdom

SUPRIYA S. VENUGOPAL, MBBS, MMed (USYD)
Dermatology Registrar, Department of Dermatology, Westmead Hospital, Westmead;
PhD Student, Department of Dermatology, St George Hospital, University of New South
Wales, Kogarah, Sydney, New South Wales, Australia

VICTORIA P. WERTH, MD
Chief, Division of Dermatology, Philadelphia Veterans Affairs Medical Center; Professor,
Department of Dermatology, University of Pennsylvania, Philadelphia, Pennsylvania

Contents

Bullous pemphigoid, the most common autoimmune blistering disease, is induced by autoantibodies against type XVII collagen. Passive transfer of IgG or IgE antibodies against type XVII collagen into animals has revealed not only the pathogenicity of these antibodies but also the subsequent immune responses, including complement activation, mast cell degranulation, and infiltration of neutrophils and/or eosinophils. In vitro studies on ectodomain shedding of type XVII collagen have also provided basic knowledge on the development of bullous pemphigoid. The pathogenic role of autoreactive CD4+ T lymphocytes in the development of the pathogenic autoantibodies to type XVII collagen should also be noted.

Bullous pemphigoid (BP) represents the most common autoimmune subepidermal blistering disease. BP typically affects the elderly and is associated with significant morbidity. It has usually a chronic course with spontaneous exacerbations. The cutaneous manifestations of BP can be extremely protean. While diagnosis of BP in the bullous stage is straightforward, in the non-bullous stage or in atypical variants of BP signs and symptoms are frequently non-specific with eg, only itchy excoriated, eczematous, papular and/or urticarial lesions that may persist for several weeks or months. Diagnosis of BP critically relies on immunopathologic examinations including direct immunofluorescence microscopy and detection of serum autoantibodies by indirect immunofluorescence microscopy or BP180-ELISA.

Autoimmune bullous diseases are associated with autoimmunity against structural components that maintain cell-cell and cell-matrix adhesion in the skin and mucous membranes. They include those where the skin blisters at the basement membrane zone and those where the skin blisters within the epidermis (pemphigus vulgaris, pemphigus foliaceus, and other subtypes of pemphigus). The variants of pemphigus are determined according to the level of intraepidermal split formation. There are 5 main variants of pemphigus: pemphigus vulgaris, pemphigus foliaceus, pemphigus erythematosus, drug-induced pemphigus, and paraneoplastic pemphigus. This review focuses only on pemphigus vulgaris.

Linear IgA disease is one of the rarer subepidermal blistering diseases. Linear IgA disease is a chronic, acquired, autoimmune blistering disease that is characterized by subepidermal blistering and linear deposition of IgA basement membrane antibodies. The disease affects both children and adults and, although there are some differences in their clinical presentations, there is considerable overlap with shared immunopathology and immunogenetics.

Dermatitis herpetiformis (DH) is characterized by chronic, itching papules, seropapules, small vesicles and, exceptionally, large blisters. The distribution of these polymorphic symptoms around the elbow, knee, buttock, and back is suggestive of the diagnosis. DH is further confirmed by the accumulation of granulocytes at the papillary dermis, resulting in a subepidermal split formation and by the presence of a unique, granular IgA precipitate in the uppermost dermis. Prognosis is predominantly determined by other autoimmune pathologies, malabsorption, or very rarely by lymphomas. Some of these diseases can be prevented by an early-onset, strict gluten-free diet, which is therefore the suggested treatment option.

Dermatitis herpetiformis (DH) is an autoimmune blistering skin disease in which antigen presentation in the gastrointestinal mucosa results in cutaneous IgA deposition and distinct, neutrophil-driven cutaneous lesions. Our findings suggest that the qualitatively different immune response to gluten in the intestinal mucosa of patients with DH results in minimal clinical symptoms, allowing the continued ingestion of gluten and the eventual development of DH. Our model may provide a new way to understand the pathogenesis of other skin diseases associated with gastrointestinal inflammation such as pyoderma gangrenosum or erythema nodosum, or explain association of seronegative inflammatory arthritis with inflammatory bowel disease.

The major treatment strategies for DH are gluten restriction or medical treatment with sulfones. Control of the cutaneous manifestations, but not the gastrointestinal changes, is rapid with dapsone. In addition to control of the cutaneous signs and symptoms of DH, dietary gluten restriction also induces improvement of gastrointestinal morphology and is possibly protective against the development of lymphoma.

John W. Frew and Dédée F. Murrell

Corticosteroids, while providing rapid remission and ongoing control of symptoms of autoimmune blistering diseases (AIBD), have numerous potentially serious acute and long-term side effects. Evidence-based medicine has reevaluated the various types of corticosteroids and forms of corticosteroid delivery in AIBD to ascertain whether any advantages of specific delivery systems or regimens exist. Careful monitoring of patients and simple preventive measures are effective in minimizing the adverse outcomes associated with their use. This article outlines the current level of evidence for corticosteroid use in AIBDs, and discusses appropriate investigations and interventions to minimize or prevent the associated adverse effects.

Volker Meyer and Stefan Beissert

Although there are no standard guidelines for the treatment of autoimmune blistering diseases, azathioprine has shown good efficacy in acquired autoimmune blistering diseases, and is well tolerated. Side effects of azathioprine normally occur in mild variants. Severe reactions are due to reduced thiopurine S-methyltransferase (TPMT) or inosine triphosphate pyrophosphohydrolase (ITPA) activity. Therefore, screening for TPMT activity should be conducted in white patients and Africans, whereas Japanese should be screened for ITPA activity before therapy with azathioprine is started. Azathioprine is clinically meaningful for the treatment of pemphigus.

Marina Eskin-Schwartz, Michael David, and Daniel Mimouni

Immunosuppressive agents such as azathioprine, cyclophosphamide, and mycophenolate mofetil (MMF) are now widely used in the treatment of autoimmune bullous diseases. This article reviews the use of MMF for the treatment of several bullous conditions, and assesses the evidence gathered from clinical trials and case series. According to numerous case series, MMF could be of value in treating refractory disease. The few randomized clinical trials conducted to date of patients with pemphigus and bullous pemphigoid report a similar efficacy for MMF to other immunosuppressants.

Evan W. Piette and Victoria P. Werth

Dapsone is used in the treatment of autoimmune bullous diseases (AIBD), a group of disorders resulting from autoimmunity directed against basement membrane and/or intercellular adhesion molecules on cutaneous and mucosal surfaces. This review summarizes the limited published data evaluating dapsone as a therapy for AIBD.

IMMUNOLOGY AND ALLERGY CLINICS OF NORTH AMERICA

Foreword

Cutaneous Immunity and Autoimmunity

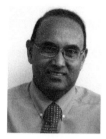

Rafeul Alam, MD, PhD
Consulting Editor

Skin is an immune system favorite. There is plenty of rationale for this favoritism. Skin serves as an environment-sensing organ for the immune system. There are immune cells that are specifically generated to address the defense and surveillance need of the skin. These cells include dermal dendritic cells, Langerhans cells, resident memory T cells, and dendritic epidermal T cells.[1,2] There are specific homing receptors for the skin, eg, cutaneous leukocyte antigen (CLA), CCR4, and CCR10. CLA+ T cells reside primarily in the skin. There are high numbers of gamma-delta T cells and NKT cells in the skin. A proper immune response against innocuous environmental agents is very important. Keratinocytes carry out this responsibility through the expression of receptors for pathogen-associated molecular patterns and release of antimicrobial peptides and pro-inflammatory cytokines. Tolerance against noninnocuous foreign antigens and self-antigens is an equally important function of the immune system. Dermal DC and CD25+Foxp3+ T cells contribute to this tolerance. How this tolerance breaks down in blistering autoimmune diseases remains still elusive.

The fundamental abnormality that characterizes blistering autoimmune skin diseases is the presence of autoantibodies against the intercellular adhesion molecules of skin.[3] Some studies also suggest a contribution from autoantibodies against nicotinic acetylcholine receptors in acantholysis.[4] The detection of autoantibodies in the skin has been the standard of diagnosis. Refinement of technology has raised enthusiasm for ELISA- and immunoblotting-based detection of these autoantibodies in the serum. There are exciting therapeutic developments in this area. They include intravenous immunoglobulin, plasmapheresis, immunoadsorption, extracorporeal photochemotherapy, biological agents such as rituximab, as well as experimental therapies such as cholinergic receptor agonists, desmoglein 3 peptides, and a p38 mitogen-activated protein kinase inhibitor. Many of these new agents are undergoing clinical trials.

Supported by NIH Grants RO1 AI091614, PPG HL 36577, and N01 HHSN272200700048C.

Immunol Allergy Clin N Am 32 (2012) xi–xii
doi:10.1016/j.iac.2012.04.014
0889-8561/12/$ – see front matter © 2012 Elsevier Inc. All rights reserved.
immunology.theclinics.com

Allergists and immunologists often see referrals for patients with skin rash. Blistering skin diseases constitute a part of these referrals. For this reason an update on blistering skin diseases would benefit not only knowledge-thirsty immunologists but also astute clinicians. This issue of the *Immunology and Allergy Clinics* presents an update on this subject from the recognized experts and leaders of the field.

Rafeul Alam, MD, PhD
Division of Allergy and Immunology
National Jewish Health and
University of Colorado Denver Health Sciences Center
1400 Jackson Street
Denver, CO 80206, USA

E-mail address:
AlamR@NJHealth.org

REFERENCES

1. Di Meglio P, Perera GK, Nestle FO. The multitasking organ: recent insights into skin immune function. Immunity 2011;35:857–69.
2. Jiang X, Clark RA, Liu L, et al. Skin infection generates non-migratory memory CD8+ TRM cells providing global skin immunity. Nature 2012;483:227–31.
3. Kasperkiewicz M, Zillikens D, Schmidt E. Pemphigoid diseases: pathogenesis, diagnosis, and treatment. Autoimmunity 2012;45:55–70.
4. Vu TN, Lee TX, Ndoye A, et al. The pathophysiological significance of nondesmoglein targets of pemphigus autoimmunity. Development of antibodies against keratinocyte cholinergic receptors in patients with pemphigus vulgaris and pemphigus foliaceus. Arch Dermatol 1998;134:971–80.

Preface

Autoimmune Diseases of the Skin

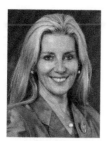

Dédée F. Murrell, MA, BMBCh, FAAD, MD, FACD
Guest Editor

There have been very few textbooks devoted to autoimmune skin diseases. If considering the definition of an autoimmune skin disease caused by autoantibody deposition in the skin, then most of these diseases manifest as blistering diseases. Unlike a textbook, where the articles may be over a year or two out of date by the time the book is published, these articles have been written in the previous 6 to 12 months and by respected leaders in the particular aspects of autoimmune blistering skin diseases (AIBD).

Experts in other areas of autoimmune disease, in particular, immunologists, will benefit from finding up-to-date information on this advancing area within dermatology. In this special issue, pathogenesis and clinical features of bullous pemphigoid are covered by Hiroshi Shimizu and his laboratory in Japan and Luca Borradori and his team in Switzerland, respectively.

Clinical features of pemphigus vulgaris is covered by Supriya Venugopal and Dédée Murrell in Sydney; linear IgA disease is covered from clinical features, diagnosis, and pathogenesis by Vanessa Venning and the team at Oxford, which stemmed from Fenella Wojnarowska's work on the subject over many years. On dermatitis herpetiformis, expert Sarolta Kárpáti from Budapest wrote about the clinical features and Russell Hall from Duke wrote on the pathogenesis and management of dermatitis herpetiformis.

Some of the drugs that are commonly used to treat AIBD are discussed in detail first by dermatologists familiar in their use for AIBD, including John Frew and Dédée Murrell on corticosteroids, Stefan Beissert from Germany on azathioprine, Daniel Mimouni from Israel on mycophenolate mofetil, Vicky Werth from the University of Pennsylvania on dapsone, Shien-Ning Chee and Dédée Murrell on intravenous immunoglobulin, and Benjamin Daniel and Dédée Murrell with Pascal Joly from Rouen, France, on rituximab. This is important because the major morbidity and mortality that these patients have (apart from the risk of blindness in mucous membrane pemphigoid) stem from the treatments themselves. It is not merely a matter of writing a prescription for oral steroids without considering what can be done from baseline to reduce the risks of significant side effects from corticosteroids.

Immunol Allergy Clin N Am 32 (2012) xiii–xiv
doi:10.1016/j.iac.2012.04.015
0889-8561/12/$ – see front matter © 2012 Elsevier Inc. All rights reserved.

immunology.theclinics.com

Hopefully this special issue will be educational for immunologists and allergists dealing with patients presenting with blistering diseases as well as scientists, family members, and the patients themselves. Understanding what is known so far about a disease leads to improved clinical practice, better research, and improved compliance with therapy.

Dédée F. Murrell, MA, BMBCh, FAAD, MD, FACD
Department of Dermatology
St George Hospital
University of New South Wales
Gray Street, Kogarah
Sydney, NSW 2217, Australia

E-mail address:
d.murrell@unsw.edu.au

Pathogenesis of Bullous Pemphigoid

Hideyuki Ujiie, MD, PhD*, Wataru Nishie, MD, PhD,
Hiroshi Shimizu, MD, PhD

KEYWORDS

- Bullous pemphigoid • Pathogenesis • Type XVII collagen
- NC16A • Animal model • IgE autoantibody

Bullous pemphigoid (BP), the most common autoimmune blistering disorder, is induced by autoantibodies against the components of the skin basement membrane zone (BMZ).[1,2] Clinically, tense blisters and erosions with itchy urticarial plaques and erythema develop on the whole body (**Fig. 1A**). Histologic examination of lesional skin reveals subepidermal blisters with inflammatory infiltration consisting of eosinophils and lymphocytes (see **Fig. 1B**). Direct immunofluorescence (IF) shows linear deposition of IgG and complement C3 at the dermal-epidermal junction (DEJ) (see **Fig. 1C**). In addition, indirect IF using the patient's sera shows linear deposition of IgG at the DEJ of normal human skin, and the autoantibodies usually deposit on the roof side of the artificial split-skin blister induced by 1M sodium chloride (see **Fig. 1D**). Immunoblotting reveals that the autoantibodies usually react with 180-kDa or 230-kDa proteins in epidermal extractions of normal human skin as candidate autoantigens. The 230-kDa protein, called BP230 or BPAG1, is a plakin family protein that was originally identified as the major antigen for BP.[3,4] BP230 is a cytoplasmic component of hemidesmosomes that enhances the linkage of keratin intermediate filaments to hemidesmosomes.[5] Although several studies have indicated that BP230 is pathogenic,[6,7] it remains unclear whether the autoantibodies against BP230 are pathogenic. The 180-kDa protein is considered to be the main pathogenic antigen in BP.

THE MAJOR PATHOGENIC ANTIGEN IN BP: TYPE XVII COLLAGEN (COL17)

Autoantibodies against the hemidesmosomal antigen of type XVII collagen (COL17, also called BP180 or BPAG2), a 180-kDa protein, are believed to induce the inflammatory process, resulting in dermal-epidermal separation. COL17 is a type II transmembrane protein that spans the lamina lucida and projects into the lamina densa of the

A version of this article was previously published in *Dermatologic Clinics 29:3*.

Financial disclosures and conflicts of interest: The authors have nothing to disclose.

Department of Dermatology, Hokkaido University Graduate School of Medicine, N-15 W-7, Kita-ku, Sapporo 060-8638, Japan

* Corresponding author.

E-mail address: h-ujiie@med.hokudai.ac.jp

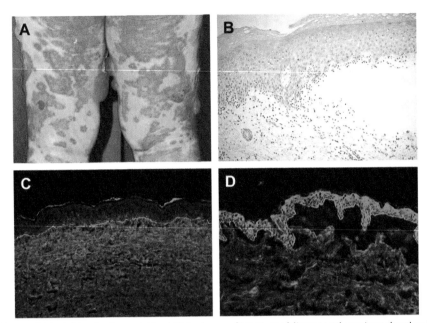

Fig. 1. Clinical, histologic, and direct IF features of BP. Tense blisters and erosions develop in itchy edematous erythema on the thighs (A). Histopathologic finding in a skin specimen taken from a tense bulla. Subepidermal blister formation associated with dermal inflammatory cell infiltration mainly of eosinophils and lymphocytes (B). Direct IF of lesional skin shows linear deposition of IgG at the DEJ (C). Indirect IF using 1M sodium chloride split skin as a substrate shows linear deposition of IgG on the roof side of the separation at the DEJ (D).

BMZ (**Fig. 2**A).[8–10] COL17 has 15 collagenous domains in the extracellular domain (see **Fig. 2**B).[11] The noncollagenous 16A (NC16A) domain in the juxtamembranous extracellular part is considered to have the major pathogenic epitope for BP (see **Fig. 2**B).[12,13] The extracellular part of COL17 is constitutively shed from the cell surface within the NC16A domain.[14]

Epitope mapping using several fragments of COL17 and enzyme-linked immunosorbent assay analysis has elucidated that sera from most patients with BP recognize NC16A.[12,15] The titer of anti-COL17 NC16A antibodies has been shown to correlate with the disease severity of BP.[16] Autoantibodies against COL17 other than its NC16A domain are also detected in BP sera. About half of the BP sera recognize the C-terminal regions of the extracellular domain of COL17, and the presence of autoantibodies against both NC16A and the C-terminal portions of COL17 seems to be associated with the clinical involvement of mucosal lesions in patients with BP.[17] Epitope spreading has been suggested as a mechanism for the generation of autoantibodies against various parts of COL17 in patients with BP.[18] Intramolecular epitope spreading within COL17 has been shown in an animal model developed by grafting human COL17-expressing transgenic (Tg) mice skin on to wild-type mice.[19] The pathogenic role of autoantibodies against COL17 other than its NC16A domain has not been fully elucidated.

Recently, precise cleavage sites within the NC16A domain of COL17 have been reported.[20] Cleavage of collagen XVII was shown to generate neoepitopes around aminoterminal cleavage sites on the shed ectodomain. It is well known that autoantibodies

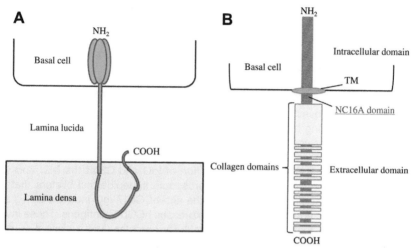

Fig. 2. The COL17 molecule in vivo. COL17 is a type II transmembrane protein that spans the lamina lucida and projects into the lamina densa of the epidermal BMZ. The extracellular domain of COL17 has at least 1 loop structure in the lamina densa in vivo (*A*). The extracellular region of COL17 involves 15 collagenous domains separated from one another by noncollagenous domains. The noncollagenous 16A (NC16A) domain, located at the membrane-proximal region of COL17, is considered to be the major pathogenic epitope for BP (*B*).

from patients with BP[21] as well as from patients with linear IgA bullous dermatosis[22] preferentially recognize the shed ectodomain of COL17, 1 explanation for which could be that these autoantibodies recognize shedding-generating neoepitopes.[20]

The pathogenicity of anti-COL17 IgG antibodies from patients with BP (BP-IgG) has been shown in vitro. BP-IgG against recombinant COL17 NC16A caused dermal-epidermal separation in cryosections of human skin when the skin was incubated with leukocytes from healthy volunteers.[23] In addition, polyclonal rabbit antibodies that target the shedding-generating neoepitopes also showed the potential to induce dermal-epidermal separation in human skin cryosections.[20] Furthermore, antibodies reacted with the nonblistering regions at the periphery of blister in patients with BP, suggesting the presence of neoepitopes in the early stage of BP that are likely to be involved in the pathogenesis of BP.[20]

Although some previous studies mentioned the pathogenic role of complement activation in BP, Iwata and colleagues[24] have reported that only BP-IgG is able to deplete the expression of COL17 in cultured normal human keratinocytes and reduce the attachment of cells from the dish in a complement-independent manner. This finding suggests that BP-IgG could reduce the content of hemidesmosomal COL17, resulting in weakness of the adhesion of hemidesmosomes to the lamina lucida.

IN VIVO STUDIES ON BP

The pathogenic role of antibodies against COL17 has been shown in a passive transfer mouse model using rabbit IgG antibodies against the murine homolog of human COL17 NC16A (murine COL17 NC14A).[25] The injected neonatal mice show skin fragility associated with the linear deposition of rabbit IgG and mouse C3 at the DEJ of their skin, and subepidermal separation with inflammatory cell infiltration; these correspond to the clinical, histologic, and immunopathologic features of BP.[25] Using this experimental BP model, Liu and colleagues revealed that subepidermal blister formation in their neonatal mouse model depends on complement activation,[26] mast cell degranulation,[27] and neutrophil infiltration.[28] These investigators also showed that the degradation of COL17 in that model depends on neutrophil elastase secreted by infiltrating neutrophils.[29]

Passive transfer of BP-IgG fails to induce a BP-like phenotype in mice, which is explained by the low similarity of the NC16A amino acid sequence between humans and mice. To further investigate the pathogenic roles of antihuman COL17 antibodies, a Tg mouse expressing human COL17 (hCOL17) cDNA driven under the control of a keratin 14 promoter was generated.[30] Olasz and colleagues[30] reported that wild-type mice grafted with hCOL17 Tg skin produce a high level of anti-hCOL17 IgG and lose the Tg skin grafts with the deposition of IgG and C3 at the DEJ and with a neutrophil infiltration, resulting in the microscopic subepidermal blisters that are observed in BP. These findings show that the anti-hCOL17 IgG induced by Tg skin grafting is pathogenic against Tg skin that expresses hCOL17 antigens. These investigators also showed that major histocompatibility complex (MHC) class II$^{-/-}$ mice grafted with Tg skin develop neither anti-hCOL17 IgG nor graft loss, indicating that MHC II and CD4$^+$ T-cell interactions are crucial for these responses.

Although these studies strongly supported the hypothesis that anti-hCOL17 IgG autoantibodies in patients with BP have pathogenic activity, such activity had not been directly shown in vivo. In 2007, Nishie and colleagues[31] confirmed this hypothesis by using the unique technique of humanization of autoantigen. First, they generated murine Col17-knockout (mCol17$^{-/-}$) mice that developed blisters and erosions on the skin, symptoms that reproduce the human disease non-Herlitz epidermolysis bullosa, which is caused by null mutations in the COL17A1 gene. By crossing Col17 knockout mice with hCOL17-expressing Tg mice, COL17-humanized (hCOL17$^{+/+}$, mCol17$^{-/-}$) mice were generated. Those COL17-humanized mice lack mCol17 but express hCOL17. Neonatal COL17-humanized mice were passively transferred with BP-IgG, which produced diffuse erythema and epidermal detachment by gentle skin friction associated with dermal-epidermal separation and inflammatory cell infiltration of neutrophils and lymphocytes (**Fig. 3**A, B). Direct IF showed linear deposition of human IgG and murine C3 at the DEJ (see **Fig. 3**C, D), which simulates the human BP phenotype. This passive transfer neonatal mouse model was the first to directly show the pathogenicity of BP-IgG in vivo.

Some studies focusing on complement activation have been performed using a neonatal COL17-humanized BP mouse model. Wang and colleagues[32] generated recombinant Fab fragments against hCOL17 NC16A from antibody repertoires of patients with BP using a phage display method. Complement activation is considered to be critical for blister formation in neonatal BP model mice.[27] Some of the recombinant Fab fragments showed marked ability to inhibit the binding of BP autoantibodies to hCOL17 and to inhibit subsequent complement activation in vitro. Those recombinant Fabs also prevented the binding of anti-COL17 NC16A antibodies to the NC16A domain in neonatal COL17-humanized mice and inhibited complement activation. Li and colleagues[33] recently generated a recombinant IgG1 monoclonal antibody against hCOL17 NC16A that can reproduce the BP phenotype in the neonatal COL17-humanized mice. These investigators introduced alanine substitutions at various C1q binding sites of the Fc region of the monoclonal antibody. Those mutated IgG antibodies failed to activate the complement in vitro and drastically lost pathogenic activity in neonatal COL17-humanized mice.[33] These 2 studies indicate that antibody-dependent complement activation is necessary for blister formation in neonatal BP model mice.

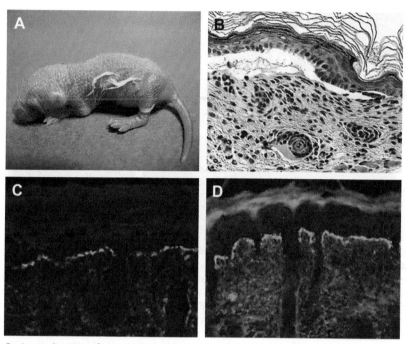

Fig. 3. A passive transfer neonatal BP model using the COL17-humanized mouse. The neonatal COL17-humanized mouse that was passively transferred with IgG affinity-purified against hCOL17 NC16A from patients with BP shows epidermal detachment by gentle skin friction at 48 hours after transfer (*A*). Lesional skin specimen shows dermal-epidermal separation and infiltration of inflammatory cells, including neutrophils and lymphocytes (*B*). Direct IF reveals linear deposition of human IgG (*C*) and murine C3 (*D*) at the DEJ.

Those passive transfer animal models show only transient disease activity. Recently, an active BP mouse model that continuously produces pathogenic IgG in vivo and that stably shows the BP phenotype has been developed using immuno-deficient $Rag-2^{-/-}$/COL17-humanized mice.[34] Adoptive transfer of splenocytes from wild-type mice immunized by the grafting of hCOL17-expressing Tg mouse skin into $Rag-2^{-/-}$/COL17-humanized mice induced continuous production of anti-hCOL17 IgG and blister formation corresponding to the clinical, histologic, and immunopatho-logic features of BP (**Fig. 4**). This study also showed that CD4+ T cells are crucial for the development of the BP phenotype in the active BP model.[34] In human BP, the presence of autoreactive CD4+ T cells has been reported, indicating the pathogenic role of CD4+ T cells in producing BP.[35–37] High frequencies of particular MHC class II alleles have been also reported.[38] These findings indicate that the autoreactive CD4+ T cells may be activated through the interaction of the specific MHC class II molecule in BP.

STUDIES ON IGE ANTIBODIES AGAINST COL17

Not only IgG but also IgE autoantibodies against COL17 are considered to be pathogenic in patients with BP.[39] The early urticarial phase of the eruptions seen in BP seems to be associated with IgE, which is based on the common knowledge of

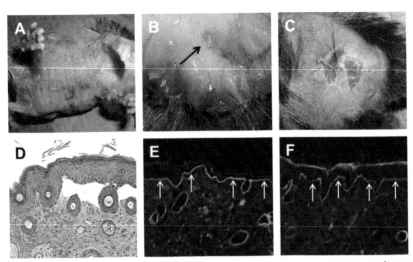

Fig. 4. Clinical, histologic, and direct IF features of an active BP mouse model. *Rag-2*$^{-/-}$/COL17-humanized mice given immunized splenocytes show large patches of hair loss associated with erythema, and erosions and crusts on the trunk and paws (*A*). Spontaneously developing blisters are also observed in the recipients (*arrow*) (*B*). Epidermal detachment by gentle friction on the trunk is observed (*C*). Histologic examination of diseased mice reveals separation between dermis and epidermis with mild inflammatory cell infiltration (*D*). Direct IF of lesional skin biopsy reveals linear deposition of mouse IgG (*arrows*) (*E*) and mouse C3 (*arrows*) (*F*) at the DEJ.

IgE-mediated degranulation of mast cells in allergic forms of urticaria.[40] Total IgE levels are increased in 70% of untreated patients with BP and IgE autoantibodies against COL17 are detected in 86% of untreated patients with BP.[41] Iwata and colleagues[42] reported that the existence of IgE autoantibodies against COL17 relates to a severe form of BP. Patients with BP with IgE against COL17 require a longer period of treatment of remission, greater amounts of corticosteroids, and more intensive treatments for remission.[42] These findings suggest that IgE autoantibodies against COL17 are associated with BP pathogenesis and disease activity.

The passive transfer models for BP using IgG against COL17 do not induce the eosinophil infiltration that is a characteristic finding in human BP.[25,31] Zone and colleagues[43] successfully reproduced the itchy erythematous lesions in engrafted human skin in SCID (severe combined immunodeficiency) mice using IgE antibodies against LABD97, a component of the shed ectodomain of hCOL17, which are generated with IgE hybridoma to the LABD97 antigen. The hybridoma was injected subcutaneously in SCID mice engrafted with human skin, and they produced IgE antibodies against LABD97 in vivo. The IgE bound to the DEJ of the engrafted human skin and induced erythema. Then, all the injected mice developed severe eosinophil infiltration and mast cell degranulation within the grafts and most of them developed histologic, but not clinically detectable, subepidermal blisters. This BP model induced by IgE antibodies reproduces the clinical and histologic findings of human BP lesions including eosinophil infiltration.

Fairley and colleagues[44] developed an experimental BP mouse model using IgE autoantibodies from patients with BP. They isolated total IgE from BP sera and injected it into human skin grafted onto athymic nude mice. Increased erythematous plaques similar to early-stage BP lesions developed in all the human skin grafts after injection of the BP IgE. Histologic examination of the lesions revealed the engorgement of blood vessels and a dermal inflammatory infiltrate composed of neutrophils, eosinophils, and degranulated mast cells. Higher doses of BP IgE autoantibodies induced histologic dermal-epidermal separation in the grafts. This study provided direct evidence of a pathogenic role for IgE autoantibodies in BP. More recently, these investigators[45] reported a case of steroid-unresponsive BP that was successfully treated with omalizumab, a humanized monoclonal antibody that inhibits IgE binding to the high-affinity receptor FcεRI, suggesting that IgE autoantibodies could be a new therapeutic target in BP.

SUMMARY

Recent studies using animal models have shown the pathogenicity of IgG and IgE antibodies against COL17 as well as the subsequent immune responses, such as complement activation, mast cell degranulation, and infiltration of inflammatory cells, including of neutrophils and/or eosinophils, although some of these responses seem to remain controversial. Moreover, in vitro studies of COL17 protein reveal the precise mechanisms of dermal-epidermal separation. The autoreactive CD4$^+$ T lymphocytes that probably serve as a commander of autoimmune reactions in BP should be further investigated, because they are a potential therapeutic target in BP.

REFERENCES

1. Bernard P, Vaillant L, Labeille B, et al. Incidence and distribution of subepidermal autoimmune bullous skin diseases in three French regions. Bullous Diseases French Study Group. Arch Dermatol 1995;13:48–52.
2. Marazza G, Pham HC, Scharer L, et al. Incidence of bullous pemphigoid and pemphigus in Switzerland: a 2-year prospective study. Br J Dermatol 2009;161: 861–8.
3. Stanley JR, Hawley-Nelson P, Yuspa SH, et al. Characterization of bullous pemphigoid antigen: a unique basement membrane protein of stratified squamous epithelia. Cell 1981;24:897–903.
4. Stanley JR, Tanaka T, Mueller S, et al. Isolation of complementary DNA for bullous pemphigoid antigen by use of patients' autoantibodies. J Clin Invest 1988;82: 1864–70.
5. Guo L, Degenstein L, Dowling J, et al. Gene targeting of BPAG1: abnormalities in mechanical strength and cell migration in stratified epithelia and neurologic degeneration. Cell 1995;81:233–43.
6. Hall RP 3rd, Murray JC, McCord MM, et al. Rabbits immunized with a peptide encoded for by the 230-kD bullous pemphigoid antigen cDNA develop an enhanced inflammatory response to UVB irradiation: a potential animal model for bullous pemphigoid. J Invest Dermatol 1993;101:9–14.
7. Kiss M, Husz S, Janossy T, et al. Experimental bullous pemphigoid generated in mice with an antigenic epitope of the human hemidesmosomal protein BP230. J Autoimmun 2005;24:1–10.
8. Diaz LA, Ratrie H 3rd, Saunders WS, et al. Isolation of a human epidermal cDNA corresponding to the 180-kD autoantigen recognized by bullous pemphigoid and herpes gestationis sera. Immunolocalization of this protein to the hemidesmosome. J Clin Invest 1990;86:1088–94.
9. Bedane C, McMillan JR, Balding SD, et al. Bullous pemphigoid and cicatricial pemphigoid autoantibodies react with ultrastructurally separable epitopes on

the BP180 ectodomain: evidence that BP180 spans the lamina lucida. J Invest Dermatol 1997;108:901–7.

10. Ishiko A, Shimizu H, Kikuchi A, et al. Human autoantibodies against the 230-kD bullous pemphigoid antigen (BPAG1) bind only to the intracellular domain of the hemidesmosome, whereas those against the 180-kD bullous pemphigoid antigen (BPAG2) bind along the plasma membrane of the hemidesmosome in normal human and swine skin. J Clin Invest 1993;91:1608–15.

11. Giudice GJ, Emery DJ, Diaz LA. Cloning and primary structural analysis of the bullous pemphigoid autoantigen BP180. J Invest Dermatol 1992;99:243–50.

12. Giudice GJ, Emery DJ, Zelickson BD, et al. Bullous pemphigoid and herpes gestationis autoantibodies recognize a common non-collagenous site on the BP180 ectodomain. J Immunol 1993;151:5742–50.

13. Zillikens D, Rose PA, Balding SD, et al. Tight clustering of extracellular BP180 epitopes recognized by bullous pemphigoid autoantibodies. J Invest Dermatol 1997;109:573–9.

14. Franzke CW, Bruckner-Tuderman L, Blobel CP. Shedding of collagen XVII/BP180 in skin depends on both ADAM10 and ADAM9. J Biol Chem 2009;284:23386–96.

15. Zillikens D, Mascaro JM, Rose PA, et al. A highly sensitive enzyme-linked immunosorbent assay for the detection of circulating anti-BP180 autoantibodies in patients with bullous pemphigoid. J Invest Dermatol 1997;109:679–83.

16. Haase C, Budinger L, Borradori L, et al. Detection of IgG autoantibodies in the sera of patients with bullous and gestational pemphigoid: ELISA studies utilizing a baculovirus-encoded form of bullous pemphigoid antigen 2. J Invest Dermatol 1998;110:282–6.

17. Hofmann S, Thoma-Uszynski S, Hunziker T, et al. Severity and phenotype of bullous pemphigoid relate to autoantibody profile against the NH2- and COOH-terminal regions of the BP180 ectodomain. J Invest Dermatol 2002;119:1065–73.

18. Di Zenzo G, Grosso F, Terracina M, et al. Characterization of the anti-BP180 autoantibody reactivity profile and epitope mapping in bullous pemphigoid patients. J Invest Dermatol 2004;122:103–10.

19. Di Zenzo G, Calabresi V, Olasz EB, et al. Sequential intramolecular epitope spreading of humoral responses to human BPAG2 in a transgenic model. J Invest Dermatol 2009;130:1040–7.

20. Nishie W, Lamer S, Schlosser A, et al. Ectodomain shedding generates Neoepitopes on collagen XVII, the major autoantigen for bullous pemphigoid. J Immunol 2010;185:4938–47.

21. Schumann H, Baetge J, Tasanen K, et al. The shed ectodomain of collagen XVII/BP180 is targeted by autoantibodies in different blistering skin diseases. Am J Pathol 2000;156:685–95.

22. Hofmann SC, Voith U, Schonau V, et al. Plasmin plays a role in the in vitro generation of the linear IgA dermatosis antigen LADB97. J Invest Dermatol 2009;129:1730–9.

23. Sitaru C, Schmidt E, Petermann S, et al. Autoantibodies to bullous pemphigoid antigen 180 induce dermal-epidermal separation in cryosections of human skin. J Invest Dermatol 2002;118:664–71.

24. Iwata H, Kamio N, Aoyama Y, et al. IgG from patients with bullous pemphigoid depletes cultured keratinocytes of the 180-kDa bullous pemphigoid antigen (type XVII collagen) and weakens cell attachment. J Invest Dermatol 2009;129:919–26.

25. Liu Z, Diaz LA, Troy JL, et al. A passive transfer model of the organ-specific autoimmune disease, bullous pemphigoid, using antibodies generated against the hemidesmosomal antigen, BP180. J Clin Invest 1993;92:2480–8.

26. Liu Z, Giudice GJ, Swartz SJ, et al. The role of complement in experimental bullous pemphigoid. J Clin Invest 1995;95:1539–44.
27. Chen R, Ning G, Zhao ML, et al. Mast cells play a key role in neutrophil recruitment in experimental bullous pemphigoid. J Clin Invest 2001;108:1151–8.
28. Liu Z, Giudice GJ, Zhou X, et al. A major role for neutrophils in experimental bullous pemphigoid. J Clin Invest 1997;100:1256–63.
29. Liu Z, Shapiro SD, Zhou X, et al. A critical role for neutrophil elastase in experimental bullous pemphigoid. J Clin Invest 2000;105:113–23.
30. Olasz EB, Roh J, Yee CL, et al. Human bullous pemphigoid antigen 2 transgenic skin elicits specific IgG in wild-type mice. J Invest Dermatol 2007;127:2807–17.
31. Nishie W, Sawamura D, Goto M, et al. Humanization of autoantigen. Nat Med 2007;13:378–83.
32. Wang G, Ujiie H, Shibaki A, et al. Blockade of autoantibody-initiated tissue damage by using recombinant fab antibody fragments against pathogenic autoantigen. Am J Pathol 2010;176:914–25.
33. Li Q, Ujiie H, Shibaki A, et al. Human IgG1 monoclonal antibody against human collagen L17 noncollagenous 16A domain induces blisters via complement activation in experimental bullous pemphigoid model. J Immunol 2010;185:7746–55.
34. Ujiie H, Shibaki A, Nishie W, et al. A novel active mouse model for bullous pemphigoid targeting humanized pathogenic antigen. J Immunol 2010;184:2166–74.
35. Budinger L, Borradori L, Yee C, et al. Identification and characterization of autoreactive T cell responses to bullous pemphigoid antigen 2 in patients and healthy controls. J Clin Invest 1998;102:2082–9.
36. Lin MS, Fu CL, Giudice GJ, et al. Epitopes targeted by bullous pemphigoid T lymphocytes and autoantibodies map to the same sites on the bullous pemphigoid 180 ectodomain. J Invest Dermatol 2000;115:955–61.
37. Thoma-Uszynski S, Uter W, Schwietzke S, et al. Autoreactive T and B cells from bullous pemphigoid (BP) patients recognize epitopes clustered in distinct regions of BP180 and BP230. J Immunol 2006;176:2015–23.
38. Delgado JC, Turbay D, Yunis EJ, et al. A common major histocompatibility complex class II allele HLA-DQB1* 0301 is present in clinical variants of pemphigoid. Proc Natl Acad Sci U S A 1996;93:8569–71.
39. Provost TT, Tomasi TB Jr. Immunopathology of bullous pemphigoid. Basement membrane deposition of IgE, alternate pathway components and fibrin. Clin Exp Immunol 1974;18:193–200.
40. Friedmann PS. Assessment of urticaria and angio-oedema. Clin Exp Allergy 1999;29(Suppl 3):109–12.
41. Dimson OG, Giudice GJ, Fu CL, et al. Identification of a potential effector function for IgE autoantibodies in the organ-specific autoimmune disease bullous pemphigoid. J Invest Dermatol 2003;120:784–8.
42. Iwata Y, Komura K, Kodera M, et al. Correlation of IgE autoantibody to BP180 with a severe form of bullous pemphigoid. Arch Dermatol 2008;144:41–8.
43. Zone JJ, Taylor T, Hull C, et al. IgE basement membrane zone antibodies induce eosinophil infiltration and histological blisters in engrafted human skin on SCID mice. J Invest Dermatol 2007;127:1167–74.
44. Fairley JA, Burnett CT, Fu CL, et al. A pathogenic role for IgE in autoimmunity: bullous pemphigoid IgE reproduces the early phase of lesion development in human skin grafted to nu/nu mice. J Invest Dermatol 2007;127:2605–11.
45. Fairley JA, Baum CL, Brandt DS, et al. Pathogenicity of IgE in autoimmunity: successful treatment of bullous pemphigoid with omalizumab. J Allergy Clin Immunol 2009;123:704–5.

Clinical Features and Practical Diagnosis of Bullous Pemphigoid

Enno Schmidt, MD, PhD[a,b,*], Rocco della Torre, MD[c],
Luca Borradori, MD[c]

KEYWORDS

- Autoantibody • BP180 • BP230 • ELISA
- Immunofluorescence microscopy

Bullous pemphigoid (BP) belongs to the group of autoimmune subepidermal blistering diseases, which are characterized by an autoantibody response directed against distinct components of the dermoepidermal junction of skin and adjacent mucous membranes. Besides BP, this group, which has overlapping clinical and immunopathologic features, also comprises pemphigoid gestationis (also called gestational pemphigoid), mucous membrane pemphigoid, linear IgA disease, anti-p200/laminin γ1 pemphigoid, and epidermolysis bullosa acquisita.

Pemphigoid diseases were first differentiated from pemphigus in 1953 by Lever[1] who described intraepidermal split formation and loss of cell adherence between keratinocytes (acantholysis) as the histopathologic hallmark of pemphigus, whereas he coined the term pemphigoid for conditions in which a subepidermal split formation was typically present. A decade later, Jordon and colleagues[2] showed that patients with BP had tissue-bound and circulating autoantibodies directed against the dermoepidermal junction. Further milestones in the understanding of BP included the

A version of this article was previously published in *Dermatologic Clinics 29:3*.

The work is dedicated to Leonie and Justus, who came into being during the preparation of this manuscript, thereby changing the life of E.S.

Conflict of Interest: E.S. has a scientific cooperation with Euroimmun AG, Lübeck. R.d.S. and L.B. have nothing to disclose.

Funding: This work was in part supported by the Schleswig-Holstein Cluster of Excellence in Inflammation Research (DFG EXC 306/1, to E.S.), by grants of the European Community's FP7 (Coordination Theme 1 HEALTH-F2-2008-200515) and the Swiss National Foundation for Scientific Research (31003A-121966 and 31003A-09811, to L.B.).

[a] Department of Dermatology, University of Lübeck, Ratzeburger Allee 160, 23538 Lübeck, Germany; [b] Comprehensive Center for Inflammation Medicine, University of Lübeck, Ratzeburger Allee 160, 23538 Lübeck, Germany; [c] Department of Dermatology, Inselspital, University Hospital of Bern, Freiburgstrasse, 3010 Bern, Switzerland
* Corresponding author.
E-mail address: enno.schmidt@uk-sh.de

immunochemical characterization of the hemidesmosomal target proteins BP180 (also called BPAG2 or type XVII collagen) and BP230 (BPAG1-e), the cloning of their genes, and the demonstration that autoantibodies to BP180 are pathogenic.[3–7]

EPIDEMIOLOGY

The incidence of BP has been estimated at between 4.5 and 14 new cases per million per year.[8–13] In a recent prospective study encompassing the entire Swiss population, the incidence was found to be 12.7 new cases per million per year.[14] These data are consistent with a recent prospective study in Lower Franconia, a well-defined region in southern Germany, where the incidence of BP was estimated to be 13.4/1 million/y.[15] A higher incidence of 42.8/1 million/y has recently been reported in Great Britain based on a data registry established on the general practitioner level. However, the British study, in which the immunopathologic criteria used were not specified, did not differentiate the various pemphigoid diseases and most likely also included bullous drug eruptions.[10] In Lower Franconia, Germany, and Great Britain the incidence of BP has considerably increased within the last 10 years (twofold and 4.8-fold, respectively),[10,15,16] an observation that may be related to either the increasing age of the general population or a better knowledge of the disease with proper diagnosis.

BP is probably the only autoimmune diseases of which the incidence increases with age. BP is typically a disease of the elderly and its diagnosis is usually made in patients aged between 75 and 81 years.[9,14,15,17–19] In the population older than 80 years of age, the incidence is 150 to 180 new patients/1 million/y.[14,15]

CLINICAL FEATURES

The name BP itself is a pleonasm. Pemphigoid is derived from Greek and means a form of blister (pemphix, blister, and eidos, form). Hence, from a purely etymologic point of view, the adjective bullous should not be added to designate the blistering in pemphigoid. However, the spectrum of clinical presentations is extremely broad (**Boxes 1** and **2**).

Characteristically, BP is an intensely pruritic eruption with widespread blister formation. In this bullous stage, vesicles and bullae develop on apparently normal or erythematous skin together with urticated and infiltrated plaques with an occasionally annular or figurate pattern (**Fig. 1**). The blisters are tense with a clear, sometimes hemorrhagic, exudate; the Nikolsky sign is negative. Pruritus, which may be invalidating, is almost constantly present.[17] Blisters are typically symmetrically distributed and may persist for several days, leaving eroded and crusted areas. Predilection sites involve the flexural aspects of the limbs and abdomen. In our own prospective Swiss cohort of patients encompassing 164 patients with BP for a 2-year period, the clinical

---

Box 1
Clinical manifestations suggestive of BP in elderly patients with chronic pruritic skin eruptions

- Papular and/or urticarial lesions
- Eczematous lesions
- Prurigo-like lesions
- Excoriations, hemorrhagic crusts
- Localized vesicles or erosions

Box 2
Unusual clinical variants of BP

- Dyshidrosiform pemphigoid
- Intertrigo-like pemphigoid
- Prurigo-nodularis-like pemphigoid
- Papular pemphigoid
- Lymphomatoid papulosis–like
- Vesicular/eczematous pemphigoid
- Erythrodermic pemphigoid
- Localized forms
  - pretibial
  - peristomal
  - umbilical
  - stump pemphigoid
  - on paralyzed body sites
  - on irradiated/traumatized body sites
- Brunsting-Perry form (variant of cicatricial pemphigoid)

---

presentation at time of diagnosis consisted of typical blisters localized on the trunk and on the extremities in about 80% of cases. In the intertriginous spaces, vegetating plaques may occur, and oral lesions develop in 10% to 20% of cases.[20] The mucosae of eyes, nose, pharynx, esophagus, and anogenital areas are rarely affected (reviewed in Refs.[21,22]).

However, before the development of tense generalized blisters, BP is typically preceded by a prodromal nonbullous phase. In this stage, diagnosis is difficult. Mild to intractable pruritus, alone or in association with excoriated, eczematous, popular, and/or urticarial lesions are found that may persist for several weeks or even months (see **Box 1**; **Fig. 2**). These unspecific skin findings may remain the only signs of the

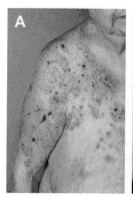
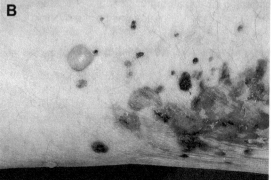

Fig. 1. Bullous pemphigoid. (*A*) Confluent urticated plaques and eczematous lesions with tense blisters on the trunk and right arm. (*B*) Close-up view.

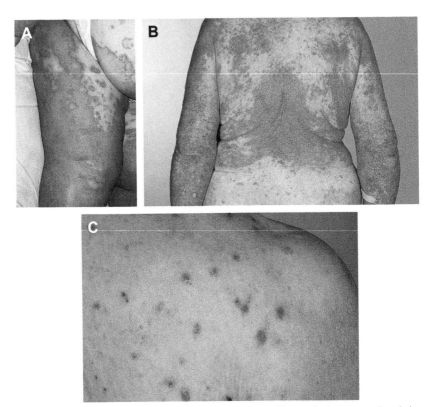

Fig. 2. Bullous pemphigoid. (*A*) Erythematous urticarial infiltrated plaques on the abdomen and legs with a figurate distribution. (*B*) Extensive eczematous and urticarial lesions on the trunk and arms. (*C*) Prurigo nodularis–like lesions and excoriated lesions on the shoulder.

disease. In this same context, several clinical variants of BP (see **Box 2**) (reviewed in Ref.[22]) have been described with a variety of different denominations, such as prurigo nodularis–like, prurigo-like,[23] erythrodermalike, ecthyma gangrenosum–like,[24] intertrigolike, and toxic epidermolysis–like lesions. Localized forms have been described confined to areas affected by radiotherapy, surgery, trauma, and burns, as well as lesions limited around stomata, hemodialysis fistulae,[25] the pretibial (**Fig. 3**) or umbilical area,[26] the palmoplantar region (mimicking dyshidrotic eczema), and the genital area.

TRIGGER FACTORS AND ASSOCIATED DISEASES

Several triggers have been implicated in the disease onset of individual patients, including trauma, burns, radiotherapy, and ultraviolet radiation. In addition, various autoimmune disorders, psoriasis, and neurologic disorders have also been described in association with BP. A large variety of drugs have been anecdotally reported to induce BP. A weak association with aldosterone antagonists and neuroleptics was found[27] and, most recently, with spironolactone and phenothiazines with aliphatic side chains.[28] Based on these data, the use of latter drugs should be carefully evaluated in BP. In 2 case-control studies including more than 1700 patients with BP and age-matched controls in Sweden and Japan, a low association with gastric cancer was identified in the Japanese cohort.[29,30] The previously described higher incidence

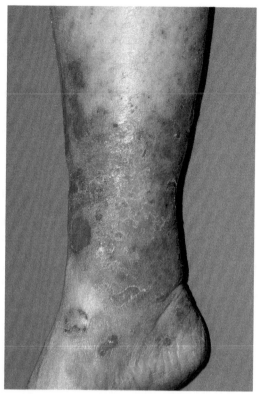

Fig. 3. Localized bullous pemphigoid: pretibial form. Postbullous erosions and eczematous lesions on the right lower leg.

of malignancies in patients with BP was probably biased by the lack of appropriate age-matched controls and the intensive work-up of affected patients in an hospital setting. Nevertheless, patients who develop BP at less than 60 years of age may be at higher risk for an underlying malignancy.[31] We usually perform an age-related cancer screen based on patient's history and clinical examination without a systematic and extensive cancer screening.

Several autoimmune disorders, such as rheumatoid arthritis, Hashimoto thyroiditis, dermatomyositis, lupus erythematosus, and autoimmune thrombocytopenia, have been reported in BP. However, a case-control study did not find any increased risk for autoimmune disorders in BP,[32] but a genetically determined susceptibility to develop autoimmune diseases is likely. BP has also been found in association with certain inflammatory dermatoses, such as psoriasis and lichen planus[33,34]; a statistically significant link has not been provided. It is conceivable that the inflammatory process at the dermoepidermal junction in these disorders raises a secondary immune response leading to autoimmunity against the target antigens of BP (epitope-spreading phenomenon).

Most recently, the association between BP and neurologic disorders has been highlighted, such as stroke (odds ratio 2.1), Parkinson disease (odds ratio 3.0 and 2.2), major cognitive impairment (odds ratio 2.2), psychiatric disorders such unipolar and bipolar disorders (odds ratio 5.3), epilepsy (odds ratio 1.7), and most strongly with multiple sclerosis (odds ratio 6.7 and 10.7).[28,35–37] These findings are particularly intriguing because some evidence has been provided suggesting that both antigens BP180 and BP230 are expressed in the central nervous system,[38–40] and mice with either target disruption of or inherited mutations in the dystonin (DST) gene encoding for various isoforms of BPAG1 (including the epithelial isoform BP230/BPAG1-e) develop severe dystonia and sensory nerve degeneration.[41]

TARGET ANTIGENS

In BP, autoantibodies recognize BP180 (also known as type XVII collagen or BP antigen 2) and BP230 (also known as BPAG1-e or BP antigen 1). These proteins are components of junctional adhesion complexes called hemidesmosomes, which are expressed in stratified and complex epithelia, such as skin, mucous membranes, and the ear, nose, and throat area. BP180 is a transmembrane glycoprotein of about 1500 amino acids. Ultrastructurally, it spans the lamina lucida before kinking back from the lamina densa into the lamina lucida (reviewed in Refs.[42,43]). The juxtamembrane domain of the extracellular portion of BP180 called NC16A was identified as the immunodominant region of BP180 in BP.[44,45] BP180 interacts with the β4 chain of α6β4 integrin, plectin, BP230, and most likely with laminin 332[46]). It provides a structural link between the intermediate filaments of the cytoskeleton and dermal collagen fibers. The importance of BP180 for the structural integrity of the skin is attested to by the observation that pathogenic mutations in its gene, COLXVII, lead to nonlethal junctional epidermolysis bullosa.[47]

In contrast, BP230 is an intracellular constituent of the hemidesmosomal plaque and belongs to the plakin family of cytolinkers. Its globular C-terminal domain mediates the anchorage of keratin filaments to the cell membrane.[46] Targeted inactivation of the DST gene encoding BP230 in mice resulted in mild skin fragility. Unexpectedly, affected mice developed neurologic defects with sensory neuron degeneration.[41] The phenotype was identical to those observed in mice suffering from dystonia musculorum, with a spontaneous mutation in the so called DST gene.[48–50] Better understanding of the phenotype of these animals has led to characterization of several tissue-specific isoforms of BP230, including at least a neuronal and a muscle-specific variant. These findings, together with the recently highlighted increased association between BP and neurologic disorders,[28,35–37] may suggest that autoimmunity to BP230 is involved in the development of neurologic diseases. Recently, mutations in the DST gene have been identified in a patient with epidermolysis bullosa exhibiting mild, localized blistering.[51]

DIAGNOSIS

Diagnosis of BP is based on a combination of clinical features and immunopathologic findings (**Fig. 4**).[43,52] In atypical and nonbullous variants, diagnosis of BP critically relies on the findings of direct immunofluorescence (IF) microscopy together with the characterization of the specificity of circulating autoantibodies and/or findings from other approaches (**Fig. 4**).

Clinical Criteria

The typical patient with BP is older than 75 years and presents with a pruritic eczematous, urticarial eruption with or without frank blistering. Mucous membranes and the face and neck region are usually not affected. In many patients, there are simply excoriated lesions. Knowledge of the wide spectrum of clinical presentations and atypical variants is important to consider the diagnosis of BP. Vaillant and colleagues[53] showed that the diagnosis of BP can be made with high specificity and sensitivity in

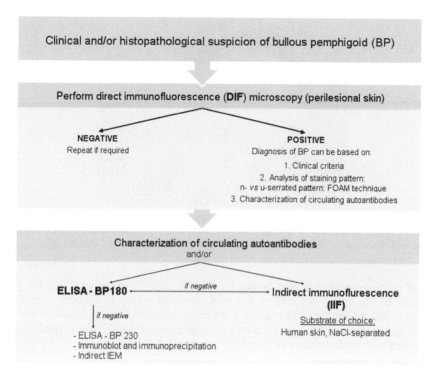

Fig. 4. Bullous pemphigoid. Diagnostic algorithm.

patients with linear immunoglobulin G (IgG) and/or C3 deposits along the dermoepidermal junction when 3 of the 4 clinical criteria are present: age greater than 70 years, absence of atrophic scars, absence of mucosal involvement, and absence of predominant bullous lesions on the neck and head.[53]

Histopathology and Immunohistochemistry

Histopathology is not essential for the diagnosis of BP. Findings may be either typical or suggestive, or at least useful, for the differential diagnosis. When BP is suspected, the biopsy specimen should ideally include a macroscopically visible vesicle, a bulla, or at least the edge of a larger bulla. Light microscopy studies of an early bulla typically reveal a subepidermal blister formation with a superficial dermal inflammatory infiltrate rich in eosinophils (**Fig. 5**) In early nonbullous phases, subepidermal clefts and eosinophilic spongiosis can be found. Recently, immunohistochemical studies have suggested that the detection of C3d deposits at the dermoepidermal junction in formalin-fixed tissue is useful for the diagnosis.[54,55]

Direct IF Microscopy

Studies of a biopsy specimen obtained from perilesional skin still represent the diagnostic gold standard. They show the presence of deposits of IgG and/or C3 along the dermoepidermal junction (**Fig. 6A**). IgM, IgE and fibrinogen may also be detected with variable frequency. The proper choice of the site for the skin biopsy is critical because lesional biopsies may give false-positive or false-negative results. Close analysis of the linear fluorescence pattern at the BMZ (n-serrated vs u-serrated pattern)[56] as well as examination of patient's skin after treatment with 1 M NaCl (referred to as salt-split

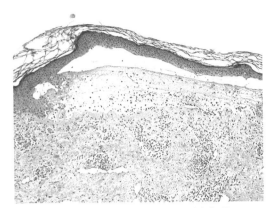

Fig. 5. Light microscopy of a fresh bulla from a patient with bullous pemphigoid (hematoxylin-eosin stain): subepidermal blister formation with discrete inflammatory infiltrate (eosinophils and neutrophils) in the blister cavity and in the dermis by light microscopy.

skin of autologous skin) is also helpful for the diagnosis[57]: In patients with BP, IgG localizes to the epidermal side of the split, whereas a dermal staining is seen in patients with anti-laminin 332 mucous membrane pemphigoid, anti-p200/laminin γ1 pemphigoid, and epidermolysis bullosa acquisita, respectively. The distribution of C3 seems less reliable than that of IgG.[58]

Indirect IF Microscopy

In up to 80% to 85% of patients, indirect IF microscopy studies show the presence of circulating IgG autoantibodies that typically bind to the epidermal side of 1M NaCl-split normal human skin, the substrate of reference (see **Fig. 6**B), differentiating BP sera from sera from patients with anti-laminin 332 mucous membrane pemphigoid, anti-p200/laminin γ1 pemphigoid, and epidermolysis bullosa acquisita, which all bind to the dermal side.[59,60] Additional circulating autoantibodies of the IgA, IgE, and IgM class can also be found. Isotype reactivity with the epidermal side of the artificial split appeared to be associated with age: sera from younger patients contained

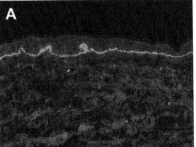
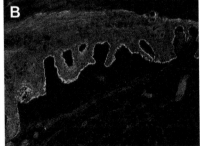

Fig. 6. (*A*) Direct immunofluorescence microscopy study of perilesional skin from a patient with bullopus pemphigoid revealed linear, continuous deposits of C3 along the dermoepidermal junction. (*B*) Indirect immunofluorescence microscopy study using NaCl-split normal human skin as a substrate. Staining of the epidermal side of the split typical for autoantibodies in bullous pemphigoid.

significantly more IgA reactivity, whereas IgG reactivity was predominantly found in older patients.[61]

Enzyme-linked Immunosorbent Assays

Enzyme-linked immunosorbent assays (ELISAs) using recombinant proteins of various portions of BP180 (such as the NC16A domain, the C-terminal portion, or its entire ecto-domain) have been found to be highly specific and sensitive.[62–73] The NC16A domain of BP180 has been identified as an immunodominant stretch in BP IgG. These anti-BP180 NC16A antibodies were found in between 75% and 90% of patients with BP[44,45,68,69,71–73] and their level correlates with the disease activity of patients with BP.[20,71,73–76] Two highly sensitive and specific ELISA systems for serum anti-BP180 antibodies are commercially available (Euroimun, Lübeck, Germany and MBL, Nagoya, Japan).[72,73]

Most patients with BP also develop, beside IgG, IgA anti-BP180 reactivity.[77] Sera from patients with linear IgA bullous disease also contain IgG and IgA antibodies against BP180,[61,77] suggesting that these 2 diseases belong to the same group of disorders. IgE reactivity against BP180 NC16A is also found in most patients with BP.[78–80] In recent studies, 10% of BP sera contained IgE but no IgG reactivity with the NC16A domain,[80] and IgE anti-BP180 antibodies were shown to contribute to tissue damage in mouse models.[81,82]

Autoantibodies against BP230, the other targeted antigen in BP, can also been detected by ELISA.[70,83–85] The globular C-terminal domain of BP230 is targeted by about 80% of the BP230-reactive BP sera.[20,86] Two ELISA kits have been commercial-ized (Euroimun and MBL) and use a recombinant C-terminal stretch of BP230, whereas, in the MBL ELISA, an N-terminal fragment is also included. Both ELISA systems are less sensitive compared with the BP180 ELISA, with anti-BP230 reactivity in only 50% to 70% of BP sera.[70,83–85] For routine analysis, a search for anti-BP230 antibodies is only helpful in patients with positive direct IF microcopy but negative BP180 ELISA reactivity.

Immunoblot and Immunoprecipitation

In the past, detection of anti-BP180 and anti-BP230 reactivity relied on immunoblot and immunoprecipitation studies using extracts of cultured keratinocytes or human epidermis,[3,5,87,88] conditioned medium of cultured human keratinocytes, as well as various recombinant forms of BP180 and BP230 produced in different expression systems.[45,66,77,78,89–91] The combination of various ELISAs with immunoblotting, as well as cell-based IF studies, allows the detection of autoantibodies in virtually all BP sera.[20,90] Currently, immunoblotting and immunoprecipitation studies are only used for investigative studies.

REACTIVITY WITH BP180 AND BP230 IN INDIVIDUALS WITHOUT BP

In a large cohort of 337 patients with various dermatologic disorders, 4.2% of the tested sera showed low positive values for BP180 (range between 9.2 and 33.1; normal, <9.0) and BP230 (range between 9.1 and 15.2; normal, <9.0), independently of age or sex.[92] Foureur and colleagues[93] confirmed this finding in a group of 138 dermatologic patients without evidence for BP. However, anti-BP180 reactivity has also been reported in patients with a variety of pruritic disorders.[94–96] At present, the detection of low-level anti-BP180 and anti-BP230 serum antibodies in patients without clinical signs of BP does not require further investigations. In patients with pruritic disorders and ELISA reactivity against BP180 or BP230, direct IF microscopy is required to differentiate between unspecific autoantibody reactivity and BP.

DIFFERENTIAL DIAGNOSIS

In our experience, BP is a great imitator. In either the nonbullous prodromal stage or in atypical presentations, it can bear close resemblance to a variety of dermatoses including localized or generalized drug reactions, contact and allergic dermatitis, prurigo, fixed urticaria, urticarial vasculitis, arthropod reactions, scabies, ecthyma, or even pityriasis lichenoides. Detailed patient history, clinical evaluation, histopathologic features, and, above all, direct immunofluorescence microscopy studies are essential to distinguish these disorders from BP. The development of specific and sensitive ELISA systems in recent years may now allow the serologic diagnosis of BP in most patients.

Diseases of the pemphigus group can be easily differentiated by distinctive clinical (positive Nikolski sign) and immunopathologic features. Mucous membrane pemphigoid is differentiated form BP by its predominant involvement of mucosal surfaces.[97] In contrast, the distinction of BP from linear IgA disease, epidermolysis bullosa acquisita, and anti-p200/laminin γ1 pemphigoid based simply on clinical and histopathologic features is usually impossible and requires direct IF microscopy (for linear IgA disease) and serologic analyses (for the last 2 entities). Lichen planus pemphigoides is clinically characterized by the presence of lichen planus lesions on otherwiese unaffected skin in addition to tense blisters. In dermatitis herpetiformis, direct IF microscopy findings, and particularly the serologic profile (presence of anti-tissue and anti-epidermal transglutaminase as well as anti-gliadin IgA antibodies) are characteristic.

PROGNOSIS AND MORTALITY

BP frequently has a chronic evolution with remissions and relapses. It is associated with significant morbidity, such as severe itch, bullous and eroded lesions, and impetiginization. The impact on the quality of life is significant. In a recent prospective study encompassing, at entry, 114 patients with BP, 47% of the 96 evaluable patients experienced a disease relapse within 1 year after cessation of therapy, confirming the recurring nature of the disease. There have been some controversies about the prognosis and mortality of BP.[98–104] It is likely that the reported diverging mortalities are related to the inclusion of populations of different mean age, in different general conditions (outpatients vs inpatients), and the use of different treatment protocols (oral corticosteroids, immunosuppressants) as well as diagnostic accuracy. For example, the 1-year mortality in 62 patients with a median age of 76 years, who were treated with methylprednisolone, dapsone, and clobetasol propionate cream, was as low as 6%,[98] whereas in a study of 312 patients with an average age of 82 years and treated by clobetasol propionate cream alone, the 1-year mortality was 39%.[104] The 1-year mortality after diagnosis of BP was reported to be 29%, 26%, 23%, and 19% in 369, 341, 223, and 869 patients with BP from Germany, France, the United States and the United Kingdom respectively.[10,18,19,103] Langan and colleagues[10] reported a 2.3-fold higher 1-year mortality risk for patients with BP compared with age-matched and sex-matched controls. In 2 large studies encompassing 369 and 177 patients, the following risk factors for lethal outcome in the first year after diagnosis were identified: (1) age greater than 82 and 80 years, respectively; (2) daily prednisolone dose of more than 37 mg after hospitalization; (3) serum albumin levels of less than 3.6 g/dL; (4) an erythrocyte sedimentation rate greater than 300 mm/h; and (5) a Karnofsky score of 40 or less.[19,102]

CONCLUDING REMARKS

Recent animal models of BP have provided unequivocal evidence for the pathogenic effect of autoantibodies to BP180 as well as novel insights into the cascade of events leading to tissue damage in BP. Despite these advances, BP still represents a clinical, diagnostic, and therapeutic challenge in our practice. The protean clinical features, the difficult diagnosis of early and atypical forms of BP, and the advanced age of affected patients with multiple comorbidities require a high degree of expertise and caution with the management of affected patients. Better knowledge of the pathophysiology of BP will hopefully facilitate the development of new immunomodulatory treatments with fewer side effects for this debilitating disease. The joint efforts by all international experts are required to improve the evaluation and treatment of these patients.

REFERENCES

1. Lever WF. Pemphigus. Medicine 1953;32:1–123.
2. Jordon RE, Beutner EH, Witebsky E, et al. Basement zone antibodies in bullous pemphigoid. JAMA 1967;200:751–6.
3. Labib RS, Anhalt GJ, Patel HP, et al. Molecular heterogeneity of the bullous pemphigoid antigens as detected by immunoblotting. J Immunol 1986;136:1231–5.
4. Diaz LA, Ratrie H 3rd, Saunders WS, et al. Isolation of a human epidermal cDNA corresponding to the 180-kD autoantigen recognized by bullous pemphigoid and herpes gestationis sera. Immunolocalization of this protein to the hemidesmosome. J Clin Invest 1990;86:1088–94.
5. Stanley JR, Hawley-Nelson P, Yuspa SH, et al. Characterization of bullous pemphigoid antigen: a unique basement membrane protein of stratified squamous epithelia. Cell 1981;24:897–903.
6. Liu Z, Diaz LA, Troy JL, et al. A passive transfer model of the organ-specific autoimmune disease, bullous pemphigoid, using antibodies generated against the hemidesmosomal antigen, BP180. J Clin Invest 1993;92:2480–8.
7. Nishie W, Sawamura D, Goto M, et al. Humanization of autoantigen. Nat Med 2007;13:378–83.
8. Bernard P, Vaillant L, Labeille B, et al. Incidence and distribution of subepidermal autoimmune bullous skin diseases in three French regions. Bullous Diseases French Study Group. Arch Dermatol 1995;131:48–52.
9. Jung M, Kippes W, Messer G, et al. Increased risk of bullous pemphigoid in male and very old patients: a population-based study on incidence. J Am Acad Dermatol 1999;41:266–8.
10. Langan SM, Smeeth L, Hubbard R, et al. Bullous pemphigoid and pemphigus vulgaris–incidence and mortality in the UK: population based cohort study. BMJ 2008;337:a180.
11. Gudi VS, White MI, Cruickshank N, et al. Annual incidence and mortality of bullous pemphigoid in the Grampian Region of North-east Scotland. Br J Dermatol 2005;153:424–7.
12. Cozzani E, Parodi A, Rebora A, et al. Bullous pemphigoid in Liguria: a 2-year survey. J Eur Acad Dermatol Venereol 2001;15:317–9.
13. Serwin AB, Bokiniec E, Piascik M, et al. Epidemiological and clinical analysis of pemphigoid patients in northeastern Poland in 2000-2005. Med Sci Monit 2007;13:CR360–4.
14. Marazza G, Pham HC, Scharer L, et al. Incidence of bullous pemphigoid and pemphigus in Switzerland: a 2-year prospective study. Br J Dermatol 2009;161:861–8.

15. Bertram F, Brocker EB, Zillikens D, et al. Prospective analysis of the incidence of autoimmune bullous disorders in Lower Franconia, Germany. J Dtsch Dermatol Ges 2009;7:434–40.
16. Zillikens D, Wever S, Roth A, et al. Incidence of autoimmune subepidermal blistering dermatoses in a region of central Germany. Arch Dermatol 1995;131: 957–8.
17. Kippes W, Schmidt E, Roth A, et al. [Immunopathologic changes in 115 patients with bullous pemphigoid]. Hautarzt 1999;50:866–72 [in German].
18. Parker SR, Dyson S, Brisman S, et al. Mortality of bullous pemphigoid: an evaluation of 223 patients and comparison with the mortality in the general population in the United States. J Am Acad Dermatol 2008;59:582–8.
19. Joly P, Benichou J, Lok C, et al. Prediction of survival for patients with bullous pemphigoid: a prospective study. Arch Dermatol 2005;141:691–8.
20. Di Zenzo G, Thoma-Uszynski S, Fontao L, et al. Multicenter prospective study of the humoral autoimmune response in bullous pemphigoid. Clin Immunol 2008; 128:415–26.
21. Liu HN, Su WP, Rogers RS 3rd. Clinical variants of pemphigoid. Int J Dermatol 1986;25:17–27.
22. Korman N. Bullous pemphigoid. J Am Acad Dermatol 1987;16:907–24.
23. Schmidt E, Sitaru C, Schubert B, et al. Subacute prurigo variant of bullous pemphigoid: autoantibodies show the same specificity compared with classic bullous pemphigoid. J Am Acad Dermatol 2002;47:133–6.
24. Geiss Steiner J, Trueb RM, Kerl K, et al. Ecthyma-gangrenosum-like bullous pemphigoid. Dermatology 2010;221:142–8.
25. Tran JT, Mutasim DF. Localized bullous pemphigoid: a commonly delayed diagnosis. Int J Dermatol 2005;44:942–5.
26. Schmidt E, Benoit S, Brocker EB. Bullous pemphigoid with localized umbilical involvement. Acta Derm Venereol 2009;89:419–20.
27. Bastuji-Garin S, Joly P, Picard-Dahan C, et al. Drugs associated with bullous pemphigoid. A case-control study. Arch Dermatol 1996;132:272–6.
28. Bastuji-Garin S, Joly P, Lemordant P, et al. Risk factors for bullous pemphigoid in the elderly: a prospective case-control study. J Invest Dermatol 2011;131:637–43.
29. Lindelof B, Islam N, Eklund G, et al. Pemphigoid and cancer. Arch Dermatol 1990;126:66–8.
30. Ogawa H, Sakuma M, Morioka S, et al. The incidence of internal malignancies in pemphigus and bullous pemphigoid in Japan. J Dermatol Sci 1995;9:136–41.
31. Bourdon-Lanoy E, Roujeau JC, Joly P, et al. [Bullous pemphigoid in young patients: a retrospective study of 74 cases]. Ann Dermatol Venereol 2005;132: 115–22 [in French].
32. Taylor G, Venning V, Wojnarowska F, et al. Bullous pemphigoid and autoimmunity. J Am Acad Dermatol 1993;29:181–4.
33. Wilczek A, Sticherling M. Concomitant psoriasis and bullous pemphigoid: coincidence or pathogenic relationship? Int J Dermatol 2006;45:1353–7.
34. Shipman AR, Cooper S, Wojnarowska F. Autoreactivity to bullous pemphigoid 180: is this the link between subepidermal blistering diseases and oral lichen planus? Clin Exp Dermatol 2011;36:267–9.
35. Langer-Gould A, Albers KB, Van Den Eeden SK, et al. Autoimmune diseases prior to the diagnosis of multiple sclerosis: a population-based case-control study. Mult Scler 2010;16:855–61.
36. Jedlickova H, Hlubinka M, Pavlik T, et al. Bullous pemphigoid and internal diseases - A case-control study. Eur J Dermatol 2010;20:96–101.

37. Langan SM, Groves RW, West J. The relationship between neurological disease and bullous pemphigoid: a population-based case-control study. J Invest Dermatol 2011;131:631–6.
38. Seppanen A, Suuronen T, Hofmann SC, et al. Distribution of collagen XVII in the human brain. Brain Res 2007;1158:50–6.
39. Chen J, Li L, Zeng Y, et al. Sera of elderly bullous pemphigoid patients with associated neurological diseases recognize bullous pemphigoid antigens in the human brain. Gerontology 2010. [Epub ahead of print].
40. Leung CL, Zheng M, Prater SM, et al. The BPAG1 locus: alternative splicing produces multiple isoforms with distinct cytoskeletal linker domains, including predominant isoforms in neurons and muscles. J Cell Biol 2001;154:691–7.
41. Guo L, Degenstein L, Dowling J, et al. Gene targeting of BPAG1: abnormalities in mechanical strength and cell migration in stratified epithelia and neurologic degeneration. Cell 1995;81:233–43.
42. Zillikens D, Giudice GJ. BP180/type XVII collagen: its role in acquired and inherited disorders or the dermal-epidermal junction. Arch Dermatol Res 1999; 291:187–94.
43. Di Zenzo G, Marazza G, Borradori L. Bullous pemphigoid: physiopathology, clinical features and management. Adv Dermatol 2007;23:257–88.
44. Giudice GJ, Emery DJ, Zelickson BD, et al. Bullous pemphigoid and herpes gestationis autoantibodies recognize a common non-collagenous site on the BP180 ectodomain. J Immunol 1993;151:5742–50.
45. Zillikens D, Rose PA, Balding SD, et al. Tight clustering of extracellular BP180 epitopes recognized by bullous pemphigoid autoantibodies. J Invest Dermatol 1997;109:573–9.
46. Borradori L, Sonnenberg A. Structure and function of hemidesmosomes: more than simple adhesion complexes. J Invest Dermatol 1999;112:411–8.
47. Fine JD, Eady RA, Bauer EA, et al. The classification of inherited epidermolysis bullosa (EB): report of the third international consensus meeting on diagnosis and classification of EB. J Am Acad Dermatol 2008;58:931–50.
48. Goryunov D, Adebola A, Jefferson JJ, et al. Molecular characterization of the genetic lesion in dystonia musculorum (dt-Alb) mice. Brain Res 2007;1140:179–87.
49. Brown A, Lemieux N, Rossant J, et al. Human homolog of a mouse sequence from the dystonia musculorum locus is on chromosome 6p12. Mamm Genome 1994;5:434–7.
50. Dalpe G, Leclerc N, Vallee A, et al. Dystonin is essential for maintaining neuronal cytoskeleton organization. Mol Cell Neurosci 1998;10:243–57.
51. Groves RW, Liu L, Dopping-Hepenstal PJ, et al. A homozygous nonsense mutation within the dystonin gene coding for the coiled-coil domain of the epithelial isoform of BPAG1 underlies a new subtype of autosomal recessive epidermolysis bullosa simplex. J Invest Dermatol 2010;130:1551–7.
52. Schmidt E, Zillikens D. Modern diagnosis of autoimmune blistering skin diseases. Autoimmun Rev 2010;10:84–9.
53. Vaillant L, Bernard P, Joly P, et al. Evaluation of clinical criteria for diagnosis of bullous pemphigoid. French Bullous Study Group. Arch Dermatol 1998;134:1075–80.
54. Pfaltz K, Mertz K, Rose C, et al. C3d immunohistochemistry on formalin-fixed tissue is a valuable tool in the diagnosis of bullous pemphigoid of the skin. J Cutan Pathol 2010;37:654–8.
55. Magro CM, Dyrsen ME. The use of C3d and C4d immunohistochemistry on formalin-fixed tissue as a diagnostic adjunct in the assessment of inflammatory skin disease. J Am Acad Dermatol 2008;59:822–33.

56. Vodegel RM, Jonkman MF, Pas HH, et al. U-serrated immunodeposition pattern differentiates type VII collagen targeting bullous diseases from other subepidermal bullous autoimmune diseases. Br J Dermatol 2004;151:112–8.

57. Domloge-Hultsch N, Bisalbutra P, Gammon WR, et al. Direct immunofluorescence microscopy of 1 mol/L sodium chloride-treated patient skin. J Am Acad Dermatol 1991;24:946–51.

58. Gammon WR, Kowalewski C, Chorzelski TP, et al. Direct immunofluorescence studies of sodium chloride-separated skin in the differential diagnosis of bullous pemphigoid and epidermolysis bullosa acquisita. J Am Acad Dermatol 1990;22:664–70.

59. Gammon WR, Briggaman RA, Inman AO 3rd, et al. Differentiating anti-lamina lucida and anti-sublamina densa anti-BMZ antibodies by indirect immunofluorescence on 1.0 M sodium chloride-separated skin. J Invest Dermatol 1984;82:139–44.

60. Kelly SE, Wojnarowska F. The use of chemically split tissue in the detection of circulating anti-basement membrane zone antibodies in bullous pemphigoid and cicatricial pemphigoid. Br J Dermatol 1988;118:31–40.

61. Mulyowa GK, Jaeger G, Kabakyenga J, et al. Autoimmune subepidermal blistering diseases in Uganda: correlation of autoantibody class with age of patients. Int J Dermatol 2006;45:1047–52.

62. Giudice GJ, Wilske KC, Anhalt GJ, et al. Development of an ELISA to detect anti-BP180 autoantibodies in bullous pemphigoid and herpes gestationis. J Invest Dermatol 1994;102:878–81.

63. Ide A, Hashimoto T, Amagai M, et al. Detection of autoantibodies against bullous pemphigoid and pemphigus antigens by an enzyme-linked immunosorbent assay using the bacterial recombinant proteins. Exp Dermatol 1995;4:112–6.

64. Zillikens D, Mascaro JM, Rose PA, et al. A highly sensitive enzyme-linked immunosorbent assay for the detection of circulating anti-BP180 autoantibodies in patients with bullous pemphigoid. J Invest Dermatol 1997;109:679–83.

65. Nakatani C, Muramatsu T, Shirai T. Immunoreactivity of bullous pemphigoid (BP) autoantibodies against the NC16A and C-terminal domains of the 180 kDa BP antigen (BP180): immunoblot analysis and enzyme-linked immunosorbent assay using BP180 recombinant proteins. Br J Dermatol 1998;139:365–70.

66. Haase C, Budinger L, Borradori L, et al. Detection of IgG autoantibodies in the sera of patients with bullous and gestational pemphigoid: ELISA studies utilizing a baculovirus-encoded form of bullous pemphigoid antigen 2. J Invest Dermatol 1998;110:282–6.

67. Hofmann S, Thoma-Uszynski S, Hunziker T, et al. Severity and phenotype of bullous pemphigoid relate to autoantibody profile against the NH2- and COOH-terminal regions of the BP180 ectodomain. J Invest Dermatol 2002;119:1065–73.

68. Mariotti F, Grosso F, Terracina M, et al. Development of a novel ELISA system for detection of anti-BP180 IgG and characterization of autoantibody profile in bullous pemphigoid patients. Br J Dermatol 2004;151:1004–10.

69. Sakuma-Oyama Y, Powell AM, Oyama N, et al. Evaluation of a BP180-NC16a enzyme-linked immunosorbent assay in the initial diagnosis of bullous pemphigoid. Br J Dermatol 2004;151:126–31.

70. Thoma-Uszynski S, Uter W, Schwietzke S, et al. BP230- and BP180-specific auto-antibodies in bullous pemphigoid. J Invest Dermatol 2004;122:1413–22.

71. Tsuji-Abe Y, Akiyama M, Yamanaka Y, et al. Correlation of clinical severity and ELISA indices for the NC16A domain of BP180 measured using BP180 ELISA kit in bullous pemphigoid. J Dermatol Sci 2005;37:145–9.

72. Sitaru C, Dahnrich C, Probst C, et al. Enzyme-linked immunosorbent assay using multimers of the 16th non-collagenous domain of the BP180 antigen for sensitive and specific detection of pemphigoid autoantibodies. Exp Dermatol 2007;16:770–7.
73. Kobayashi M, Amagai M, Kuroda-Kinoshita K, et al. BP180 ELISA using bacterial recombinant NC16a protein as a diagnostic and monitoring tool for bullous pemphigoid. J Dermatol Sci 2002;30:224–32.
74. Schmidt E, Obe K, Brocker EB, et al. Serum levels of autoantibodies to BP180 correlate with disease activity in patients with bullous pemphigoid. Arch Dermatol 2000;136:174–8.
75. Feng S, Wu Q, Jin P, et al. Serum levels of autoantibodies to BP180 correlate with disease activity in patients with bullous pemphigoid. Int J Dermatol 2008; 47:225–8.
76. Amo Y, Ohkawa T, Tatsuta M, et al. Clinical significance of enzyme-linked immunosorbent assay for the detection of circulating anti-BP180 autoantibodies in patients with bullous pemphigoid. J Dermatol Sci 2001;26:14–8.
77. Kromminga A, Scheckenbach C, Georgi M, et al. Patients with bullous pemphigoid and linear IgA disease show a dual IgA and IgG autoimmune response to BP180. J Autoimmun 2000;15:293–300.
78. Dopp R, Schmidt E, Chimanovitch I, et al. IgG4 and IgE are the major immunoglobulins targeting the NC16A domain of BP180 in bullous pemphigoid: serum levels of these immunoglobulins reflect disease activity. J Am Acad Dermatol 2000;42:577–83.
79. Iwata Y, Komura K, Kodera M, et al. Correlation of IgE autoantibody to BP180 with a severe form of bullous pemphigoid. Arch Dermatol 2008;144:41–8.
80. Messingham KA, Noe MH, Chapman MA, et al. A novel ELISA reveals high frequencies of BP180-specific IgE production in bullous pemphigoid. J Immunol Methods 2009;346:18–25.
81. Zone JJ, Taylor T, Hull C, et al. IgE basement membrane zone antibodies induce eosinophil infiltration and histological blisters in engrafted human skin on SCID mice. J Invest Dermatol 2007;127:1167–74.
82. Fairley JA, Burnett CT, Fu CL, et al. A pathogenic role for IgE in autoimmunity: bullous pemphigoid IgE reproduces the early phase of lesion development in human skin grafted to nu/nu mice. J Invest Dermatol 2007;127:2605–11.
83. Kromminga A, Sitaru C, Hagel C, et al. Development of an ELISA for the detection of autoantibodies to BP230. Clin Immunol 2004;111:146–52.
84. Yoshida M, Hamada T, Amagai M, et al. Enzyme-linked immunosorbent assay using bacterial recombinant proteins of human BP230 as a diagnostic tool for bullous pemphigoid. J Dermatol Sci 2006;41:21–30.
85. Tampoia M, Lattanzi V, Zucano A, et al. Evaluation of a new ELISA assay for detection of BP230 autoantibodies in bullous pemphigoid. Ann N Y Acad Sci 2009;1173:15–20.
86. Skaria M, Jaunin F, Hunziker T, et al. IgG autoantibodies from bullous pemphigoid patients recognize multiple antigenic reactive sites located predominantly within the B and C subdomains of the COOH-terminus of BP230. J Invest Dermatol 2000;114:998–1004.
87. Mueller S, Klaus-Kovtun V, Stanley JR. A 230-kD basic protein is the major bullous pemphigoid antigen. J Invest Dermatol 1989;92:33–8.
88. Bernard P, Didierjean L, Denis F, et al. Heterogeneous bullous pemphigoid antibodies: detection and characterization by immunoblotting when absent by indirect immunofluorescence. J Invest Dermatol 1989;92:171–4.

89. Marinkovich MP, Taylor TB, Keene DR, et al. LAD-1, the linear IgA bullous dermatosis autoantigen, is a novel 120-kDa anchoring filament protein synthesized by epidermal cells. J Invest Dermatol 1996;106:734–8.

90. Schmidt E, Kromminga A, Mimietz S, et al. A highly sensitive and simple assay for the detection of circulating autoantibodies against full-length bullous pemphigoid antigen 180. J Autoimmun 2002;18:299–309.

91. Tanaka M, Hashimoto T, Amagai M, et al. Characterization of bullous pemphigoid antibodies by use of recombinant bullous pemphigoid antigen proteins. J Invest Dermatol 1991;97:725–8.

92. Wieland CN, Comfere NI, Gibson LE, et al. Anti-bullous pemphigoid 180 and 230 antibodies in a sample of unaffected subjects. Arch Dermatol 2010;146: 21–5.

93. Foureur N, Mignot S, Senet P, et al. [Correlation between the presence of type-2 anti-pemphigoid antibodies and dementia in elderly subjects with no clinical signs of pemphigoid]. Ann Dermatol Venereol 2006;133:439–43 [in French].

94. Jedlickova H, Racovska J, Niedermeier A, et al. Anti-basement membrane zone antibodies in elderly patients with pruritic disorders and diabetes mellitus. Eur J Dermatol 2008;18:534–8.

95. Feliciani C, Caldarola G, Kneisel A, et al. IgG autoantibody reactivity against bullous pemphigoid (BP) 180 and BP230 in elderly patients with pruritic dermatoses. Br J Dermatol 2009;161:306–12.

96. Hofmann SC, Tamm K, Hertl M, et al. Diagnostic value of an enzyme-linked immunosorbent assay using BP180 recombinant proteins in elderly patients with pruritic skin disorders. Br J Dermatol 2003;149:910–2.

97. Chan LS, Ahmed AR, Anhalt GJ, et al. The first international consensus on mucous membrane pemphigoid: definition, diagnostic criteria, pathogenic factors, medical treatment, and prognostic indicators. Arch Dermatol 2002;138:370–9.

98. Schmidt E, Kraensel R, Goebeler M, et al. Treatment of bullous pemphigoid with dapsone, methylprednisolone, and topical clobetasol propionate: a retrospective study of 62 cases. Cutis 2005;76:205–9.

99. Colbert RL, Allen DM, Eastwood D, et al. Mortality rate of bullous pemphigoid in a US medical center. J Invest Dermatol 2004;122:1091–5.

100. Joly P, Benichou J, Saiag P, et al. Response to: mortality rate of bullous pemphigoid in a US medical center. J Invest Dermatol 2005;124:664–5.

101. Bystryn JC, Rudolph JL. Why is the mortality of bullous pemphigoid greater in Europe than in the US? J Invest Dermatol 2005;124:xx–xxi.

102. Roujeau JC, Lok C, Bastuji-Garin S, et al. High risk of death in elderly patients with extensive bullous pemphigoid. Arch Dermatol 1998;134:465–9.

103. Rzany B, Partscht K, Jung M, et al. Risk factors for lethal outcome in patients with bullous pemphigoid: low serum albumin level, high dosage of glucocorticosteroids, and old age. Arch Dermatol 2002;138:903–8.

104. Joly P, Roujeau JC, Benichou J, et al. A comparison of two regimens of topical corticosteroids in the treatment of patients with bullous pemphigoid: a multicenter randomized study. J Invest Dermatol 2009;129:1681–7.

Diagnosis and Clinical Features of Pemphigus Vulgaris

Supriya S. Venugopal, MBBS, MMed[a,b],
Dédée F. Murrell, MA, BMBCh, FAAD, MD, FACD[b,*]

KEYWORDS

• Pemphigus vulgaris • Desmoglein 3 • Diagnosis

CLINICAL PRESENTATION OF PEMPHIGUS VULGARIS

Autoimmune bullous diseases are associated with autoimmunity against structural components that maintain cell-cell and cell-matrix adhesion in the skin and mucous membranes.[1] They include those where the skin blisters at the basement membrane zone (bullous pemphigoid, herpes gestationis, mucous membrane pemphigoid, linear immunoglobulin (Ig)A dermatosis, epidermolysis bullosa acquisita, bullous lupus, and dermatitis herpetiformis) and those where the skin blisters within the epidermis (pemphigus vulgaris [PV], pemphigus foliaceus [PF], and other subtypes of pemphigus).

Because of the considerable overlap in the clinical presentation of these conditions, diagnosis of autoimmune bullous skin conditions can be challenging. Detection of tissue-bound and circulating serum autoantibodies and characterization of their molecular specificity is an important modality for diagnosis. In the past decade, there have been several advances in diagnostic modalities for autoimmune bullous skin conditions.

Pemphigus, a word derived from the Greek word "pemphix" meaning bubble or blister, is a life-threatening autoimmune blistering disease characterized by intraepithelial blister formation.[2–4] Damage to intercellular adhesion structures, desmogleins, are the target of circulating autoantibodies resulting in the hallmark of this condition, acantholysis.[5,6] Acantholysis may result in the development of the Tzanck phenomenon, which is the rounding of single epidermal cells caused by the loss of cell-cell attachment.

A version of this article was previously published in *Dermatologic Clinics 29:3*.

Financial Disclosure/Conflict of Interest Statement: The authors of this article have no financial disclosures or conflict of interest to express.

[a] Department of Dermatology, Westmead Hospital, Westmead, Sydney, NSW, Australia; [b] Department of Dermatology, St George Hospital, University of New South Wales, Ground Floor, James Laws House, Gray Street, Kogarah, Sydney, NSW 2217, Australia

* Corresponding author.

E-mail address: d.murrell@unsw.edu.au

Immunol Allergy Clin N Am 32 (2012) 233–243

doi:10.1016/j.iac.2012.04.003

0889-8561/12/$ – see front matter © 2012 Elsevier Inc. All rights reserved.

EPIDEMIOLOGY

The incidence of pemphigus is approximately 1 in 100,000 people. Pemphigus vulgaris is the most common variant of pemphigus with an incidence of 0.1 to 0.5 per 100,000 population and higher among Jewish patients.[7] In India, Malaysia, China, and the Middle East, pemphigus vulgaris accounts for 70% of all pemphigus cases and may be the most common autoimmune blistering disease.[8–10]

Various environmental and pharmacologic etiological factors have been reported in pemphigus. These factors include medications, pesticides, malignancy, ultraviolet radiation, and stress.[11–18]

Foods containing an allium, phenol, thiol, or urushiol group have also been reported to trigger pemphigus.[19,20]

Pathogenesis

PV is an autoimmune condition that is more likely to develop in patients with HLA types after certain triggers. PV is associated with several autoantibodies. The main autoantibodies target the desmosomal protein, desmoglein 3 (dsg3), a 130-kDa glycoprotein cadherin.[5] Later, there is secondary development of antibodies to another desmosomal cadherin, desmogleins 1, which is a 160-kDa glycoprotein dsg1 antigen, when the skin is involved.[21] Further potential target antigens in PV are acetylcholine receptors on keratinocytes.[22–24] Pincelli's group has shown that apoptosis pathways are triggered early in PV and are followed by desmosomal endocytosis.[25,26] In addition, David Rubenstein's group has shown that the signaling molecule p38 is rapidly phosphorylated when PV IgG is added to human keratinocytes and that inhibiting p38 blocks dsg3 endocytosis, keratin retraction, and actin reorganization. P38 is phosphorylated in the skin of neonatal mice tested with either PV or PF IgG. P38 inhibitors block blistering in both the PV and PF passive transfer mouse models. Similarly, p38 is phosphorylated in the skin of human patients with PV and PF.[27,28]

PV is strongly associated with the HLA serotypes HLA-DR4 and HLA-DR6.[29] 48% of healthy relatives of patients with PV had low levels of autoantibody and the inheritance of autoantibody positivity was linked to the DR4 and DR6 haplotype. Although population studies report differing prevalences of alleles in various ethnic groups, greater than 95% of patients with PV possess one or both of these haplotypes.[30] In 2006, Lee and colleagues[30] concluded that in the non-Jewish population, 8 alleles were positively associated and 1 allele was negatively associated with PV. The 2 candidate alleles most likely to contribute to disease susceptibility in the Non-Jewish population included DRB1*0402 and DQB1*0503. DRB1*0402 was determined to be the sole allele likely to confer susceptibility to PV in Ashkenazi Jewish patients.

CLINICAL FEATURES
Clinical Presentation

The variants of pemphigus are determined according to the level of intraepidermal split formation. There are 5 main variants of pemphigus: pemphigus vulgaris, pemphigus foliaceus, pemphigus erythematosus, drug-induced pemphigus, and paraneoplastic pemphigus. This review focuses only on PV.

Patients suffering from PV present with oral erosions and then subsequently develop cutaneous involvement.[31,32] Mucosal erosions usually precede the cutaneous manifestations of the disease and often result in a protracted course of misdiagnosis with conditions, such as aphthous ulceration. In some cases, oral ulceration may be the only manifestation of the disease. The mucosal surfaces that may be involved include the oropharynx, esophagus, conjunctiva, nasal, larynx, urethra, vulva, and cervix.[33–38]

Cutaneous involvement may be localized or generalized. Skin lesions have a predilection for the trunk, groins, axillae, scalp, face, and pressure points (**Figs. 1–4**).[39] Flaccid blisters develop on these sites and may coalesce; these blisters eventually rupture and result in painful erosions. PV usually presents in adults and can affect anywhere in the body but predominantly affects the buccal and labial mucosa (**Fig. 5**). This condition is characterized by Nikolsky's sign; the direct Nikolsky is when the application of slight pressure on a blister results in extension of the blistering to adjacent skin and the indirect Nikolsky is when rubbing on clinically normal skin causes shearing. These signs are not always 100% reliable for the diagnosis of PV, but they are suggestive if present.[40]

Other more rare clinical manifestations include nail dystrophy, paronychia, subungual hematomas, and neonatal pemphigus vulgaris.[41,42]

DIFFERENTIAL DIAGNOSIS

Patients are often treated for multiple other blistering conditions before the diagnosis of pemphigus vulgaris is made with diagnostic investigations, in particular a skin or mucosal biopsy for DIF.

The differentials for mucosal lesions include stomatitis secondary to herpes simplex virus; aphthous ulcers; lichen planus; paraneoplastic pemphigus; or autoimmune disease, such as lupus erythematosus or dermatitis herpetiformis. Differentials for cutaneous involvement include other autoimmune blistering skin conditions, such as pemphigus foliaceus, pemphigus vegetans, IgA pemphigus, paraneoplastic pemphigus,

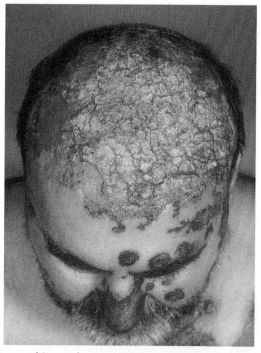

Fig. 1. Patient with pemphigus vulgaris presenting with crusted erosions on his scalp and face.

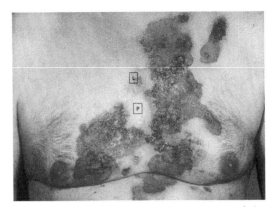

Fig. 2. Crusted, superficial erosions on the chest and abdomen of the same patient with pemphigus vulgaris. Boxed *L* indicates an appropriate site for a lesional biopsy for routine histology and boxed *P* indicates a site that is good for the perilesional biopsy for direct immunofluorescence.

bullous pemphigoid, linear IgA disease, erythema multiforme, Grover disease, and Hailey-Hailey disease.

There are a variety of blistering conditions that must be taken into consideration when suspecting that patients have pemphigus vulgaris. The etiology of blistering diseases may be broadly divided into autoimmune, infective, or inflammatory.

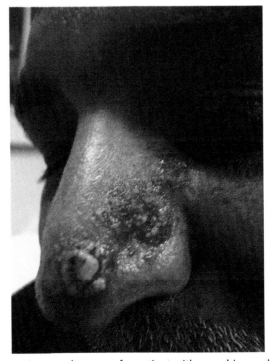

Fig. 3. Vegetative erosions on the nose of a patient with pemphigus vulgaris.

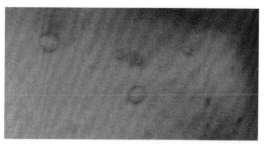

Fig. 4. Some tense and flaccid, well-circumscribed bullae and superficial erosions on the abdomen of a young woman with pemphigus vulgaris.

DIAGNOSIS

The diagnosis of PV can be made using 4 major criteria:

1. Clinical findings
2. Light microscopic findings
3. Direct immunofluorescence findings
4. Indirect immunofluorescence findings.[4,43]

The clinical findings assisting in the diagnosis of PV, a potentially life-threatening autoimmune vesiculobullous disorder, include nonscarring, fragile vesicles, and bullae involving the mucosae with varying cutaneous involvement.

The biopsies should be carefully performed on lesional and perilesional skin. The most recent, untreated lesion is the most preferable site for biopsy. At the edge of a blister (lesional) is the best site for hematoxylin and eosin (H+E) analysis to discern the presence and level of blistering or acantholysis (see **Fig. 2**). The type, density, and level of inflammatory infiltrate in conjunction with the direct immunofluorescence findings assist in making the diagnosis of pemphigus vulgaris. Lesional biopsies for H+E can be transported in formalin.

Perilesional biopsies taken within 2 cm of active blistering (see **Fig. 2**) should be taken for DIF analysis and transported in normal saline if they can get to the laboratory straight away for the best results[44] or Michel's medium otherwise. These characteristically show netlike, intercellular staining with IgG, C3, IgM, or IgA (discussed in the next section).

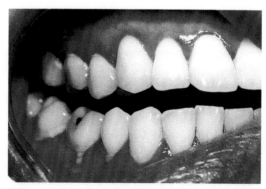

Fig. 5. Superficial, diffuse gingival erosions in a patient with pemphigus vulgaris. (*Courtesy of* Dr Schifter, Skin and Cancer Foundation, Westmead, Sydney.)

Patients with isolated mucosal disease should have lesional and perilesional mucosal biopsies performed for H+E and DIF to confirm the diagnosis of pemphigus vulgaris in conjunction with biopsies of cutaneous lesions, if clinically warranted.

HISTOPATHOLOGY

PV is usually characterized by suprabasalar loss of adhesion leaving a single layer of basal keratinocytes attached to the dermoepidermal basement membrane (tombstone pattern). This characteristic is distinguished from PF, which is associated with a more superficial split formation in the subcorneal layer. Histologic findings in PV lesions on hematoxylin and eosin demonstrate suprabasalar acantholysis and infiltration with predominantly neutrophils and eosinophils (**Fig. 6**). The early findings of pemphigus may be subtle and include suprabasalar acantholysis associated with a mild, superficial mixed inflammatory infiltrate, including some eosinophils. These changes can also be present in more developed lesions (see **Fig. 6**).

On direct immunofluorescence, IgG or C3 binding to the intercellular cement substance in the mid-lower or entire epidermis of perilesional skin or mucosa is characteristic (**Fig. 7**).[45–48]

Desmoglein 3[5] and desmoglein 1[21] are the targets for autoantibodies in PV and PF, respectively. Tissue-bound IgG, C3, IgM, or IgA in a characteristic netlike intercellular distribution pattern within the epidermis is demonstrated on direct immunofluorescence microscopy (see **Fig. 7**). Anti-dsg1 and anti-dsg3 antibodies predominantly belong to the IgG4 subclass.[49–52] Anti-IgA and IgE subclass antibodies have also been detected. Patients with predominantly mucosal involvement have antibodies only against dsg3; however, a significant proportion of mucosal-dominant disease will also have dsg1 autoantibodies.[53,54] The phenotypic presentation of pemphigus vulgaris with respect to mucosal and generalized cutaneous involvement has been attributed to the presence of desmoglein 3 and desmoglein 1 autoantibodies, respectively.[55–62]

Indirect immunofluorescence microscopy reveals the presence of serum autoantibodies against desmosomal antigens. Pemphigus sera show a characteristic netlike intercellular staining of IgG with human skin as a substrate. Other substrates, such as monkey esophagus, guinea pig esophagus or rat bladder epithelium, may be used in the diagnosis of paraneoplastic pemphigus.[63]

Enzyme-linked immunosorbent assay (ELISA) has provided higher sensitivity and specificity in making the diagnosis of pemphigus subtypes.[64] ELISA results can be used to determine pemphigus vulgaris disease activity and be used for longitudinal

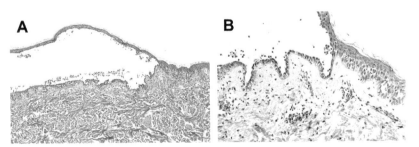

Fig. 6. Hematoxylin and eosin findings of an acute lesion of pemphigus vulgaris showing suprabasal acantholysis (*A, B*). (*From* Weedon D, Strutton G, Rubin AI. The vesiculobullous reaction pattern. In: Weedon D, editor. Weedon's Skin Pathology. 3rd edition. Philadelphia: Churchill-Livingston; 2010; with permission.)

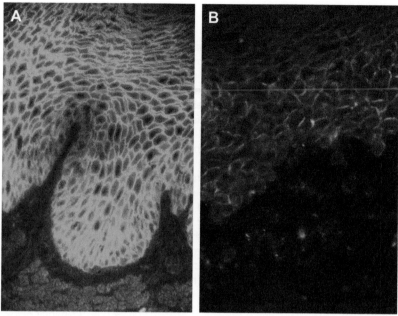

Fig. 7. Direct immunofluorescence results in a patient with pemphigus vulgaris showing intercellular staining with IgG (A) and C3 (B). (*Courtesy of* Professor Kossard, Skin and Cancer Foundation, Darlinghurst, Sydney.)

monitoring of treatment response. Antibodies can be detected in patients without clinical signs of pemphigus and can be found in patients with staphylococcal scalded skin,[65] penicillin adverse drug reactions,[66] toxic epidermolysis necrosis,[67] and burns.[68] In addition, patients with blood group O who have antibodies to blood groups A and B may give low false positives on indirect immunofluorescence testing,[69] which is avoided by preabsorbing their sera with these blood group antigens.

In active PV, immunoblot analysis with recombinant dsg3 demonstrated that anti-dsg3 of the IgG4, IgA, and IgE subtypes predominate; however, chronic remittent PV is characterized by IgG1 and IgG4 autoantibodies.[50,53]

DISEASE ACTIVITY CATEGORIZATION

The Consensus Statement on Disease Endpoints and Therapeutic Response for Pemphigus[70] divides pemphigus disease activity into the following categories:

- Early endpoints
    Baseline
    Control of disease activity
    End of consolidation phase
- Late endpoints
    Complete remission off therapy
    Complete remission on therapy
        Minimal therapy
        Minimal adjuvant therapy
        Partial remission off therapy
        Partial remission on minimal therapy

- Relapse/flare
- Treatment failure.

Early endpoints provide a useful clinical indicator for clinicians regarding the commencement of differing treatment regimes. The *baseline* is classified as the day that the treating practitioner initiates treatment. *Control of disease activity* is defined as the time at which there is cessation of new lesions in conjunction with the healing of preexisting lesions. In the majority of cases the expected time period in this stage is weeks. The *end of the consolidation phase* is the time period in which no new lesions have developed over a minimum period of 2 weeks. This phase is also characterized by the healing of most lesions, and most medical practitioners would consider the weaning of steroids.

Late endpoints of disease activity may be reached with or without therapy. *Complete remission off therapy* is characterized by the absence of new lesions over a 2-month period after cessation of therapy. *Minimal therapy* constitutes treatment with less than or equal to 10 mg/day of prednisone or the equivalent or the use of minimal adjuvant therapy for a duration of at least 2 months. *Minimal adjuvant therapy* comprises of half the dose required to be defined as treatment failure. *Partial remission off therapy* is classified as development of lesions after cessation of treatment that heal within 1 week without treatment. Patients must be off systemic therapy for 2 months to be classified in this category. Patients may suffer a partial remission on minimal therapy when they develop new lesions that heal within 1 week while receiving minimal therapy. Topical steroids also constitute minimal therapy.

A *relapse/flare* is defined by the development of 3 or more new lesions that persist without healing for greater than 1 week or by the extension of preexisting established lesions. Treatment failure results when there is no change in disease activity despite treatment on therapeutic doses of systemic steroids and other agents whose doses and durations were agreed by international consensus.[70]

ACKNOWLEDGMENTS

This article was supported in part by the University of NSW Postgraduate Awards for Dr Venugopal's PhD studies with Dedee Murrell.

REFERENCES

1. Mihai S, Sitaru C. Immunopathology and molecular diagnosis of autoimmune bullous diseases. J Cell Mol Med 2007;11(3):462–81.
2. Lever WF. Pemphigus. Medicine 1953;32:1–123.
3. Huilgol SC, Black MM. Management of the immunobullous disorders. II. Pemphigus. Clin Exp Dermatol 1995;20:283–93.
4. Hertl M. Humoral and cellular autoimmunity in autoimmune bullous skin disorders. Int Arch Allergy Immunol 2000;122:91–100.
5. Amagai M, Klaus-Kovtun V, Stanley JR. Auto-Ab against a novel epithelial cadherin in pemphigus vulgaris, a disease of cell adhesion. Cell 1991;67:869–77.
6. Bedane C, Prost C, Thomine E, et al. Binding of autoantibodies is not restricted to desmosomes in pemphigus vulgaris: comparison of 14 cases of pemphigus vulgaris and 10 cases of pemphigus foliaceus studied by western immunoblot and immunoelectron microscopy. Arch Dermatol Res 1996;288:343–52.
7. Ahmed AR, Yunis EJ, Khatri K. Major histocompatibility complex haplotype studies in Ashkenazi Jewish patients with pemphigus vulgaris. Proc Natl Acad Sci U S A 1991;87:7658–62.

8. Wilson C, Wojnarowska F, Mehra NK, et al. Pemphigus in Oxford, UK, and New Delhi, India: a comparative study of disease characteristics and HLA antigens. Dermatology 1994;189(Suppl 1):108–10.
9. Adam BA. Bullous diseases in Malaysia: epidemiology and natural history. Int J Dermatol 1992;31:42–5.
10. Chams-Davatchi C, Valikhani M, Daneshpazhooh M, et al. Pemphigus: analysis of 1209 cases. Int J Dermatol 2005;44:470–6.
11. Mashiah J, Brenner S. Medical pearl: First step in managing pemphigus–addressing the etiology. J Am Acad Dermatol 2005;53(4):706–7.
12. Brenner S, Mashiah J, Tamir E, et al. Pemphigus: an acronym for a disease with multiple etiologies. Skinmed 2003;2:163–7.
13. Brenner S, Bialy-Golan A, Ruocco V. Drug-induced pemphigus. Clin Dermatol 1998;163:393–7.
14. Goldberg I, Kashman Y, Brenner S. The induction of pemphigus by phenol drugs. Int J Dermatol 1999;38:888–92.
15. Brenner S, Wolf R, Ruocco V. Contact pemphigus: a subgroup of induced pemphigus. Int J Dermatol 1994;33:843–5.
16. Brenner S, Bar-Nathan EA. Pemphigus vulgaris triggered by emotional stress. J Am Acad Dermatol 1984;11:524–5.
17. Brenner S, Tur E, Shapiro J, et al. Pemphigus vulgaris: environmental factors. Occupational, behavioral, medical, and qualitative food frequency questionnaire. Int J Dermatol 2001;40:562–9.
18. Jacobs SE. Pemphigus erythematosus and ultraviolet light. A case report. Arch Dermatol 1965;91:139–41.
19. Brenner S, Ruocco V, Wolf R, et al. Pemphigus and dietary factors. In vitro acantholysis by allyl compounds of the genus Allium. Dermatology 1995;190: 197–202.
20. Tur E, Brenner S. Diet and pemphigus. In pursuit of exogenous factors in pemphigus and fogo selvagem. Arch Dermatol 1998;134:1406–10.
21. Emery DJ, Diaz LA, Fairley LA, et al. Detection and characterization of pemphigus foliaceus autoantibodies that react with the desmoglein-1 ectodomain. J Invest Dermatol 1995;104:323–8.
22. Grando SA. Autoimmunity to keratinocyte acetylcholine receptors in pemphigus. Dermatology 2000;201(4):290–5.
23. Sison-Fonacier L, Bystryn JC. Heterogeneity of pemphigus vulgaris antigens. Arch Dermatol 1987;123:1507–10.
24. Vu TN, Lee TX, Ndoye A, et al. The pathophysiological significance of nondesmoglein targets of pemphigus autoimmunity. Development of antibodies against keratinocyte cholinergic receptors in patients with pemphigus vulgaris and pemphigus foliaceus. Arch Dermatol 1998;134(8):971–80.
25. Grando SA, Bystyrn JC, Chernyvavsky AI, et al. Apoptolysis: novel mechanism of skin blistering in pemphigus vulgaris linking the apoptotoc pathways to basal cell shrinkage and suprabasal acantholysis. Exp Dermatol 2009;18(9):764–70.
26. Berkowitz P, Hu P, Warren S, et al. p38MAPK inhibition prevents disease in pemphigus vulgaris mice. Proc Natl Acad Sci U S A 2006;103:12855–60.
27. Berkowitz P, Chua M, Liu Z, et al. Autoantibodies in the autoimmune disease pemphigus foliaceus induce blistering via p38 mitogen-activated protein kinase-dependent signaling in the skin. Am J Pathol 2008;173:1628–36.
28. Szafer F, Brautbar C, Tzfoni E, et al. Detection of disease-specific restriction fragment length polymorphisms in pemphigus vulgaris linked to the DQw1 and DQw3 alleles of the HLA-D region. Proc Natl Acad Sci U S A 1987;84:6542.

29. Todd JA, Acha-Orbea H, Bell JI, et al. A molecular basis for MHC class II–associated autoimmunity. Science 1988;240:1003.
30. Lee E, Lendas KA, Chow S, et al. Disease relevant HLA class II alleles isolated by genotypic, haplotypic, and sequence analysis in North American Caucasians with pemphigus vulgaris. Hum Immunol 2006;67(1-2):125–39.
31. Meurer M, Millns JL, Rogers RS III, et al. Oral pemphigus vulgaris. A report of ten cases. Arch Dermatol 1977;113:1520–4.
32. Sirois DA, Fatahzadeh M, Roth R, et al. Diagnostic patterns and delays in pemphigus vulgaris: experience with 99 patients. Arch Dermatol 2000;136:1569–70.
33. Hodak E, Kremer I, David M, et al. Conjunctival involvement in pemphigus vulgaris: a clinical, histopathological and immunofluorescence study. Br J Dermatol 1990;123:615–20.
34. Hale EK, Bystryn JC. Laryngeal and nasal involvement in pemphigus vulgaris. J Am Acad Dermatol 2001;44:609–11.
35. Lurie R, Trattner A, David M, et al. Esophageal involvement in pemphigus vulgaris: report of two cases and review of the literature. Dermatologica 1990;181:233–6.
36. Trattner A, Lurie R, Leiser A, et al. Esophageal involvement in pemphigus vulgaris: a clinical, histologic, and immunopathologic study. J Am Acad Dermatol 1991;24:223–6.
37. Marren P, Wojnarowska F, Venning V, et al. Vulvar involvement in autoimmune bullous diseases. J Reprod Med 1993;38:101–7.
38. Sagher F, Bercovici B, Romem R. Nikolsky sign on cervix uteri in pemphigus. Br J Dermatol 1974;90:407–11.
39. Korman N. Pemphigus. J Am Acad Dermatol 1988;18:1219–38.
40. Uzun S, Durdu M. The specificity and sensitivity of Nikolsky sign in the diagnosis of pemphigus. J Am Acad Dermatol 2006;54:411–5.
41. Berker DD, Dalziel K, Dawber RP, et al. Pemphigus associated with nail dystrophy. Br J Dermatol 1993;129:461–4.
42. Kolivras A, Gheeraert P, Andre J. Nail destruction in pemphigus vulgaris. Dermatology 2003;206:351–2.
43. Mutasim DF. Autoimmune bullous diseases: diagnosis and management. Dermatol Nurs 1999;11:15–21.
44. Vodegel RM, de Jong MC, Meijer HJ, et al. Enhanced diagnostic immunofluorescence using biopsies transported in saline. BMC Dermatol 2004;4:10.
45. Ahmed AR, Graham J, Jordan RE, et al. Pemphigus: current concepts. Ann Intern Med 1980;92:396–405.
46. Lever WF. Pemphigus and pemphigoid. J Am Acad Dermatol 1979;1:2–31.
47. Scully C. A review of mucocutaneous disorders affecting the mouth and lips. Ann Acad Med Singapore 1999;28:704–7.
48. Scott JE, Ahmed AR. The blistering diseases. Med Clin North Am 1998;82:1239–83.
49. Ding X, Diaz LA, Fairley JA, et al. The anti-desmoglein 1 autoantibodies in pemphigus vulgaris sera are pathogenic. J Invest Dermatol 1999;112:739–43.
50. Kricheli D, David M, Frusic-Zlotkin M, et al. The distribution of pemphigus vulgaris-IgG subclasses and their reactivity with desmoglein 3 and 1 in pemphigus patients and their first-degree relatives. Br J Dermatol 2000;143:337–42.
51. Ayatollahi M, Joubeh S, Mortazavi H, et al. IgG4 as the predominant autoantibody in sera from patients with active state of pemphigus vulgaris. J Eur Acad Dermatol Venereol 2004;18:241–2.

52. David M, Katzenelson V, Mimouni D, et al. The distribution of pemphigus vulgaris-IgG subclasses in patients with active disease. J Eur Acad Dermatol Venereol 2006;20:232.

53. Spaeth S, Riechers R, Borradori L, et al. IgG, IgA and IgE autoantibodies against the ectodomain of desmoglein 3 in active pemphigus vulgaris. Br J Dermatol 2001;144:1183–8.

54. Mentink LF, de Jong MCJM, Kloosterhuis GJ, et al. Coexistence of IgA antibodies to desmogleins 1 and 3 in pemphigus vulgaris, pemphigus foliaceus and para-neoplastic pemphigus. Br J Dermatol 2007;156:635–41.

55. Amagai M, Tsunoda K, Zillikens D, et al. The clinical phenotype of pemphigus is defined by the anti-desmoglein autoantibody profile. J Am Acad Dermatol 1999; 40:167–70.

56. Jamora MJJ, Jiao D, Bystryn JC. Antibodies to desmoglein 1 and 3, and the clinical phenotype of pemphigus vulgaris. J Am Acad Dermatol 2003;48:976–7.

57. Miyagawa S, Amagai M, Iida T, et al. Late development of antidesmoglein 1 antibodies in pemphigus vulgaris: correlation with disease progression. Br J Dermatol 1999;141:1084–7.

58. Amagai M. Towards a better understanding of pemphigus autoimmunity. Br J Dermatol 2000;143:237–8.

59. Harman KE, Gratian MJ, Bhogal BS, et al. A study of desmoglein 1 autoantibodies in pemphigus vulgaris: racial differences in frequency and the association with a more severe phenotype. Br J Dermatol 2000;143:343–8.

60. Ding X, Aoki V, Mascaro JM Jr, et al. Mucosal and mucocutaneous (generalized) pemphigus vulgaris show distinct autoantibody profiles. J Invest Dermatol 1997; 109:592–6.

61. Harman KE, Seed PT, Gratian MJ, et al. The severity of cutaneous and oral pemphigus is related to desmoglein 1 and 3 antibody levels. Br J Dermatol 2001; 144:775–80.

62. Olszewska M, Gerlicz Z, Blaszczyk M. Cutaneous pemphigus vulgaris. J Eur Acad Dermatol Venereol 2007;21:698–9.

63. Jiao D, Bystryn JC. Sensitivity of indirect immunofluorescence, substrate specificity and immunoblotting in the diagnosis of pemphigus. J Am Acad Dermatol 1997;37:211–6.

64. Ishii K, Amagai M, Hall RP, et al. Characterization of autoantibodies in pemphigus using antigen-specific enzyme linked immunosorbent assays with baculovirus expressed recombinant desmogleins. J Immunol 1997;159:2010–7.

65. Anzai H, Stanley JR, Amagai M. Production of low titers of anti-desmoglein 1 IgG autoantibodies in some patients with staphylococcal scalded skin syndrome. J Invest Dermatol 2006;126:2139–41.

66. Fellner MJ, Mark AS. Penicillin- and ampicillin-induced pemphigus vulgaris. Int J Dermatol 1980;19:392–3.

67. Ahmed A, Workman A. Anti-intercellular substance antibody: presence in serum of 14 patients without pemphigus. Arch Dermatol 1983;119:17–21.

68. Thivolet J, Beyvin A. Recherche par immunofluorescence d'anticorps seriques vis-vis des constituants de l'epiderme chez les brutes. Experientia 1968;24:945–6.

69. Lee FJ, Silvestrini R, Fulcher DA. False positive intercellular cement substance antibodies due to group A/B red cell antibodies: frequency and approach. Pathology 2010;42(6):574–6.

70. Murrell DF, Amagai M, Barnadas MA, et al. Consensus statement on definitions of disease endpoints and therapeutic response for pemphigus. J Am Acad Dermatol 2008;58(6):1043–6.

Linear IgA Disease: Clinical Presentation, Diagnosis, and Pathogenesis

Vanessa A. Venning, BMBCh, DM, FRCP

KEYWORDS

- Linear IgA disease • LAD
- Chronic bullous dermatosis of childhood • CBDC

DEFINITION

Linear IgA disease (LAD) is a chronic, acquired, autoimmune blistering disease. It is characterized by subepidermal blistering and linear deposition of immunoglobulin A (IgA) basement membrane antibodies. The disease affects both children and adults and, although there are some differences in their clinical presentations, there is considerable overlap with shared immunopathology and immunogenetics.[1]

DEMOGRAPHICS AND GENETIC BACKGROUND

LAD is one of the rarer subepidermal blistering diseases, with an incidence of only 0.5 per 10^6 in western Europe. It is commoner in other parts of the world, including China, southeast Asia, and Africa, where there is a higher frequency of childhood disease.[2–4] Although LAD can come on at any age, there are 2 peaks of onset, 1 in early childhood and the other after the age of 60 years. Most children present as toddlers or preschool children, although a few have presented as neonates or in later childhood and in their teens.[1,5] Although it can affect young adults, there is a second peak of onset after the age of 60 years. The sex incidence is about equal, or there may be a slight excess of female patients.

There is a strong association between LAD and the extended autoimmune haplotype HLA-B8, HLA-CW7, HLA-DR3 in British and black South African patients, and possession of this haplotype is associated with an early disease onset. This extended haplotype is in linkage disequilibrium with an activating allele of tumor necrosis factor (TNF), and this association exists in patients with LAD and seems to worsen prognosis and prolong the disease.[6]

A version of this article was previously published in *Dermatologic Clinics 29:3*.
Department of Dermatology, Churchill Hospital, Old Road, Oxford OX3 7LJ, UK
E-mail address: vanessa.venning@orh.nhs.uk

Immunol Allergy Clin N Am 32 (2012) 245–253
doi:10.1016/j.iac.2012.04.004
0889-8561/12/$ – see front matter © 2012 Elsevier Inc. All rights reserved.

CLINICAL FEATURES

Children with LAD show differences in clinical presentation compared with adults, reflected in the common usage of the term chronic bullous disease of childhood, although the immunopathology of the childhood and adult diseases are the same.

Chronic Bullous Disease of Childhood

The typical presentation is a small child with an acute episode of blistering with variable symptoms of mild pruritus to severe burning. The first attack is usually more severe than later relapses. The face and perineal area are commonly affected with lesions around the mouth and eyes, including the eyelids or on the lower abdomen vulva, thighs, and buttocks (**Fig. 1**). Blistering on the genitalia may be mistaken for sexual abuse. The lesions may spread to the abdomen and limbs, including the hands and feet. Lesions comprise urticated plaques that frequently assume annular or polycyclic patterns, with blistering around the edge producing the so-celled string-of-pearls sign (**Fig. 2**). Blisters may become large or even hemorrhagic.

Mucosal lesions are common, with oral ulcers and erosions, nasal stuffiness or bleeding, and conjunctivitis.[1]

Differential diagnosis

In young children, bullous impetigo may resemble the initial lesions. Genetic epidermolysis bullosa is often present at birth and is also differentiated from LAD by the family history. Bullous papular urticaria rarely affects the face or genital region and is usually of short duration. Childhood bullous pemphigoid may resemble LAD.

LAD in Adults

The disease usually starts abruptly but may be insidious, with variable pruritus or a burning sensation. The trunk is almost always involved but lesions on the face, scalp, and limbs, including the hands and feet, are also common. The lesions comprise urticated plaques and papules with vesicles and blisters arising either from normal skin or from the urticated areas (**Fig. 3**). The distinctive annular and string-of-pearls grouping of blisters around the edge are less common than in children. Some cases of LAD, in particular drug-related cases, have resembled other disorders, including erythema multiforme, toxic epidermal necrolysis, and morbilliform rash without blisters.[7,8]

Mucosal involvement is common with oral ulcers and erosions. Hoarseness may indicate pharyngeal involvement. There is often nasal stuffiness and crusting, and eyes are often sore or gritty. Involvement of the genitals and also the vagina can occur.

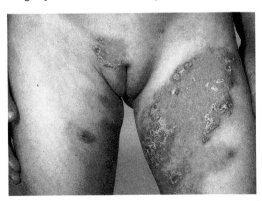

Fig. 1. LAD in childhood: blistering around the margins of annular and polycyclic lesions.

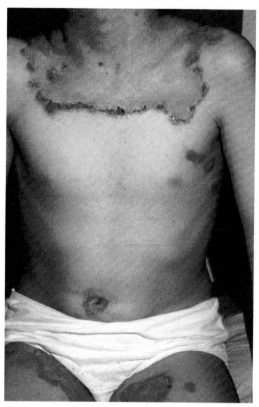

Fig. 2. LAD in childhood: blistering around the margins of annular and polycyclic lesions.

Differential diagnosis

The adult disease is frequently confused with bullous pemphigoid in most cases, and less often with atypical erythema multiforme, nodular prurigo with excoriations, and dermatitis herpetiformis. Histology is helpful and direct immunofluorescence (IMF) is essential for diagnosis.

LAD: TRIGGERS AND DISEASE ASSOCIATIONS

Drugs

Most cases start spontaneously but drug-induced LAD is well recognized. Vancomycin is the drug most frequently implicated, diclofenac and other nonsteroidal antiinflammatory drugs being less commonly reported, as well as single cases with a large range of other drugs.[7,9–12]

Skin Trauma

Skin injury including burns have been associated with triggering disease onset.[1,13,14]

Malignant Disease

Adults with LAD have an increased incidence of lymphoproliferative disorders that develop even after remission of the skin disease.[14–16] There are several case reports of other malignancies, of which bladder and renal cancer are commonest.[17–19]

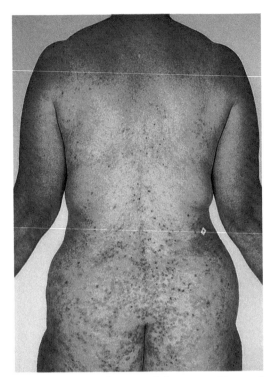

Fig. 3. LAD in an adult: extensive involvement of the torso with papulovesicular rash.

Gastrointestinal Disease

LAD has been associated with both ulcerative colitis and Crohn disease in small numbers of patients.[20,21] Patients with LAD were originally believed to have dermatitis herpetiformis. It is now clear that these 2 IgA-mediated diseases are distinct. LAD shows no association with gluten-sensitive enteropathy and does not respond to dietary gluten exclusion.[22–24]

CLINICAL COURSE AND PROGNOSIS

Most patients respond well to treatment with dapsone or other sulfone drugs, antiinflammatory antibiotics, and topical steroids,[1] This will be covered in more detail in the article by Ng and Venning in the next issue. After an initial acute attack, the disease may wax and wane slightly, with subsequent flares usually being less severe than the first. In most patients, the disease remits during the course of a few years (3–6 years) and treatment can be discontinued.[1,25] Most children remit before puberty, although it occasionally persists into adult life.[26] In general LAD does not cause scarring. A small number children and adults have exceptionally severe mucosal disease that progresses to cicatrizing conjunctivitis and even blindness.[27–29] This rare subgroup is best regarded as having mucous membrane pemphigoid in accordance with the 2002 International Consensus on Mucous Membrane Pemphigoid: Definition and Diagnostic Criteria.[27]

DIAGNOSIS

The diagnosis of LAD may be supported by histopathogy but is only confirmed by IMF studies.

Histopathology

The histologic features are not diagnostic for the condition. The blisters are subepidermal but the cellular infiltrate is variable. Some cases show eosinophil predominance suggestive of bullous pemphigoid. In others, the appearances are more in keeping with dermatitis herpetiformis with neutrophils predominating and even dermal papillary microabscesses. Others show subepidermal blisters with entirely nonspecific features.

IMF

IMF studies are essential for diagnosis. Direct IMF should be performed on clinically uninvolved skin. The back is a suitable site and is a good practical choice for biopsy in a child. Forearm skin gives lower pickup rates of positive results.[28]

On direct IMF, there is linear deposition of IgA along the basement membrane zone and, in some cases, other immunoreactants, immunoglobulin G (IgG), immunoglobulin M, or C3 are also seen.[1] In rare cases, a granular linear pattern of IgA at the basement membrane zone is seen.[29]

Indirect IMF for IgA basement membrane zone antibodies is more often positive in children (about 75%) than adults (about 30%).[1] The titers are usually low, on the order of 1:5 or 1:10, but occasionally much higher. The use as substrate of normal human skin split through the lamina lucida by incubation in saline increases the sensitivity and gives additional information as to the site of the target antigen. Most sera are roof binding, a few are floor binding, and a smaller number show a mixed pattern. Blister fluid is a suitable alternative to serum for indirect IMF testing and may be easier to obtain in a child.[30]

The presence of IgG autoantibodies on direct or indirect IMF causes problems with disease definition, occurs in both children and adults, and has been called mixed immunobullous disease. In most cases, the patients have had a clinical picture compatible with LAD and a good response to dapsone or sulfonamides. The exact position of dual responders is unclear but, for practical purposes, the patients are best managed as LAD.[31–33]

Immunoblotting

Immunoblotting of linear IgA sera may pick up a variety of target antigens, in keeping with the multiple localizations found using IMF with split skin. Using an epidermal extract for immunoblotting, the positivity rate for IgA is higher than with IMF and is positive in about 83% of adult sera and 64% of children. IgG antibodies may also be detected in more than 50% of adults and children.[34]

PATHOGENESIS

There is indirect evidence for the pathogenicity of the IgA antibodies. In an in vitro model, IgA binding caused splitting of skin in culture and binding of neutrophils to the basement membrane zone.[35] An animal model has demonstrated that linear IgA bullous disease sera passively transferred to severe combined immunodeficient mice with human skin grafts are capable of promoting neutrophil infiltration and basement membrane vesiculation.[36]

Using split skin as a substrate for IMF, most sera bind to the epidermal side of the split, implying an antigen associated with hemidesmosomes or the upper lamina lucida; a minority bind to the dermal aspect of the artificial blister suggesting a lower lamina lucida or dermal antigen, and a few sera have a combined pattern. In keeping with the IMF findings, immunoelectron microscopy (IEM) studies have shown that the immunoreactants and target antigens are either associated with the hemidesmo-somes, within the lamina lucida, in the subbasal lamina zone, or in a mirror-image pattern on each side of the lamina densa.[37,38]

TARGET ANTIGENS

In keeping with both the IMF and IEM findings, the IgA antibody response in LAD in children and adults is heterogeneous, being directed at several different target anti-gens within the adhesion complex, and most sera have more than 1 target antigen.

The major target antigen is BP180/collagen XVII, a key structural component of the dermoepidermal adhesion complex (**Fig. 4**). It has an intracellular globular domain where its NH2 terminal interacts with the NH2 terminal of BPAg1 (BP230) and other hemidesmosomal components.[39] The long, extracellular, collagenous domain of collagen XVII traverses the lamina lucida in the region of the anchoring filaments and its COOH terminal embeds into the lamina densa. Part of the extracellular portion of the collagen XVII molecule is physiologically shed and is also further degraded by proteolytic action to produce extracellular fragments, molecular weight 120 kDa and 97 kDa respectively. Ectodomain shedding seems to generate neoepitopes in collagen XVII, possibly by conformational changes in the molecule.

Most sera in LAD (in both adults and children) target part or all of the collagen XVII molecule, and T cell responses to it have also been shown.[40] Epitope mapping of the sera has produced variable results[34,41–43] but it seems that sera preferentially react with the shed ectodomain of collagen XVII or its fragment and less with its full-length form. The juxtamembranous NC16A domain collagen XVII, an important immunodomi-nant epitope in both bullous and mucous membrane pemphigoid, is also a target for IgA antibodies in LAD, frequently in conjunction with other antigenic targets.

The intracellular BP230, originally described as the major antigen in bullous pemphi-goid,[34] is also targeted by IgA antibodies, more commonly in adult than childhood LAD

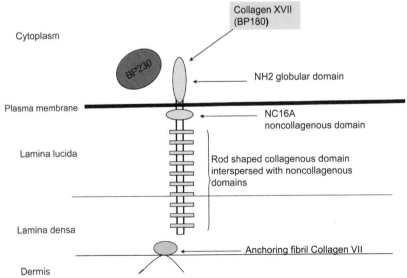

Fig. 4. Collagen XVII and other components of the dermoepidermal junction adhesion complex that may be target antigens in LAD. The NC16A domain may be a target epitope and is also the site through which enzymatic cleavage takes place to produce the shed ectodomain and neoantigens.

sera. A unique antigen, LAD285, has a molecular weight of 285 kDa and has been found in patients whose sera have both dermal and epidermal binding on IMF testing using split skin. Collagen VII, a component of the anchoring fibril, is a rare antigen. Unlike classic epidermolysis bullosa acquisita, in which there is anti–collagen VII IgG, LAD is almost never associated with a mechanobullous scarring phenotype. There are also other unidentified dermal antigens.[41]

The detection of multiple antigens by IgA suggests that there is a primary disease-provoking epitope with spread of the immune response to other epitopes on the same or adjacent molecules. Multiple target antigens occur more commonly in adults than in children, possibly reflecting more prolonged antigenic stimulation.[34] In contrast with the heterogeneity of the IgA antibody response, binding of IgG autoantibodies to multiple antigens is rare and the role of the IgG response in the development and spread of the immune response in LAD is unknown.

REFERENCES

1. Wojnarowska F, Marsden RA, Bhogal B, et al. Chronic bullous disease of childhood, childhood cicatricial pemphigoid, and linear IgA disease of adults. A comparative study demonstrating clinical and immunopathologic overlap. J Am Acad Dermatol 1988;19:792–805.
2. Adam BA. Bullous diseases in Malaysia: epidemiology and natural history. Int J Dermatol 1992;31:42–5.
3. Aboobaker J, Wojnarowska FT, Bhogal B, et al. Chronic bullous dermatosis of childhood–clinical and immunological features seen in African patients. Clin Exp Dermatol 1991;16:160–4.
4. Jin P, Shao C, Ye G. Chronic bullous dermatoses in China. Int J Dermatol 1993;32: 89–92.
5. Kishida Y, Kameyama J, Nei M, et al. Linear IgA bullous dermatosis of neonatal onset: case report and review of the literature. Acta Paediatr 2004;93:850–2.
6. Collier PM, Wojnarowska F, Welsh K, et al. Adult linear IgA disease and chronic bullous disease of childhood: the association with human lymphocyte antigens Cw7, B8, DR3 and tumour necrosis factor influences disease expression. Br J Dermatol 1999;141:867–75.
7. Dellavalle RP, Burch JM, Tayal S, et al. Vancomycin-associated linear IgA bullous dermatosis mimicking toxic epidermal necrolysis. J Am Acad Dermatol 2003;48: S56–7.
8. Billet SE, Kortuem KR, Gibson LE, et al. A morbilliform variant of vancomycin-induced linear IgA bullous dermatosis. Arch Dermatol 2008;144:774–8.
9. Collier PM, Wojnarowska F. Drug-induced linear immunoglobulin A disease. Clin Dermatol 1993;11:529–33.
10. Palmer RA, Ogg G, Allen J, et al. Vancomycin-induced linear IgA disease with autoantibodies to BP180 and LAD285. Br J Dermatol 2001;145:816–20.
11. Camilleri M, Pace JL. Linear IgA bullous dermatosis induced by piroxicam. J Eur Acad Dermatol Venereol 1998;10:70–2.
12. Bouldin MB, Clowers-Webb HE, Davis JL, et al. Naproxen-associated linear IgA bullous dermatosis: case report and review. Mayo Clin Proc 2000;75:967–70.
13. Girao L, Fiadeiro T, Rodrigues JC. Burn-induced linear IgA dermatosis. J Eur Acad Dermatol Venereol 2000;14:507–10.
14. Godfrey K, Wojnarowska F, Leonard J. Linear IgA disease of adults: association with lymphoproliferative malignancy and possible role of other triggering factors. Br J Dermatol 1990;123:447–52.

15. Jacyk WK, Nagel GJ, van der Hoven AE. Linear IgA dermatosis and Hodgkin's lymphoma–report of a case in an African and review of the literature. J Dermatol 1990;17:633–7.
16. Usmani N, Baxter KF, Child JA, et al. Linear IgA disease in association with chronic lymphocytic leukaemia. Br J Dermatol 2004;151:710–1.
17. McEvoy MT, Connolly SM. Linear IgA dermatosis: association with malignancy. J Am Acad Dermatol 1990;22:59–63.
18. van der Waal RI, van de Scheur MR, Pas HH, et al. Linear IgA bullous dermatosis in a patient with renal cell carcinoma. Br J Dermatol 2001;144:870–3.
19. Rodenas JM, Herranz MT, Tercedor J, et al. Linear IgA disease in a patient with bladder carcinoma. Br J Dermatol 1997;136:257–9.
20. Paige DG, Leonard JN, Wojnarowska F, et al. Linear IgA disease and ulcerative colitis. Br J Dermatol 1997;136:779–82.
21. Birnie AJ, Perkins W. A case of linear IgA disease occurring in a patient with colonic Crohn's disease. Br J Dermatol 2005;153:1050–2.
22. Sachs JA, Leonard J, Awad J, et al. A comparative serological and molecular study of linear IgA disease and dermatitis herpetiformis. Br J Dermatol 1988; 118:759–64.
23. Leonard JN, Griffiths CE, Powles AV, et al. Experience with a gluten free diet in the treatment of linear IgA disease. Acta Derm Venereol 1987;67:145–8.
24. Leonard JN, Haffenden GP, Unsworth DJ, et al. Evidence that the IgA in patients with linear IgA disease is qualitatively different from that of patients with dermatitis herpetiformis. Br J Dermatol 1984;110:315–21.
25. Marsden RA, McKee PH, Bhogal B, et al. A study of benign chronic bullous dermatosis of childhood and comparison with dermatitis herpetiformis and bullous pemphigoid occurring in childhood. Clin Exp Dermatol 1980;5:159–76.
26. Burge S, Wojnarowska F, Marsden A. Chronic bullous dermatosis of childhood persisting into adulthood. Pediatr Dermatol 1988;5:246–9.
27. Chan LS, Ahmed AR, Anhalt GJ, et al. The First International Consensus on Mucous Membrane Pemphigoid: definition, diagnostic criteria, pathogenic factors, medical treatment, and prognostic indicators. Arch Dermatol 2002;138: 370–9.
28. Collier PM, Wojnarowska F, Millard PR. Variation in the deposition of the antibodies at different anatomical sites in linear IgA disease of adults and chronic bullous disease of childhood. Br J Dermatol 1992;127:482–4.
29. Leonard JN, Haffenden GP, Ring NP, et al. Linear IgA disease in adults. Br J Dermatol 1982;107:301–16.
30. Zhou S, Wakelin SH, Allen J, et al. Blister fluid for the diagnosis of subepidermal immunobullous diseases: a comparative study of basement membrane zone autoantibodies detected in blister fluid and serum. Br J Dermatol 1998;139: 27–32.
31. Powell J, Kirtschig G, Allen J, et al. Mixed immunobullous disease of childhood: a good response to antimicrobials. Br J Dermatol 2001;144:769–74.
32. Sheridan AT, Kirtschig G, Wojnarowska F. Mixed immunobullous disease: is this linear IgA disease? Australas J Dermatol 2000;41:219–21.
33. Viglizzo G, Cozzani E, Nozza P, et al. A case of linear IgA disease in a child with IgA and IgG circulating antibodies directed to BPAg2. Int J Dermatol 2007;46:1302–4.
34. Allen J, Wojnarowska F. Linear IgA disease: the IgA and IgG response to the epidermal antigens demonstrates that intermolecular epitope spreading is associated with IgA rather than IgG antibodies, and is more common in adults. Br J Dermatol 2003;149:977–85.

35. Hendrix JD, Mangum KL, Zone JJ, et al. Cutaneous IgA deposits in bullous diseases function as ligands to mediate adherence of activated neutrophils. J Invest Dermatol 1990;94:667–72.

36. Zone JJ, Egan CA, Taylor TB, et al. IgA autoimmune disorders: development of a passive transfer mouse model. J Investig Dermatol Symp Proc 2004;9:47–51.

37. Bhogal B, Wojnarowska F, Marsden RA, et al. Linear IgA bullous dermatosis of adults and children: an immunoelectron microscopic study. Br J Dermatol 1987; 117:289–96.

38. Prost C, De Leca AC, Combemale P, et al. Diagnosis of adult linear IgA dermatosis by immunoelectronmicroscopy in 16 patients with linear IgA deposits. J Invest Dermatol 1989;92:39–45.

39. Hopkinson SB, Baker SE, Jones JC. Molecular genetic studies of a human epidermal autoantigen (the 180-kD bullous pemphigoid antigen/BP180): identification of functionally important sequences within the BP180 molecule and evidence for an interaction between BP180 and alpha 6 integrin. J Cell Biol 1995;130:117–25.

40. Lin MS, Fu CL, Olague-Marchan M, et al. Autoimmune responses in patients with linear IgA bullous dermatosis: both autoantibodies and T lymphocytes recognize the NC16A domain of the BP180 molecule. Clin Immunol 2002;102:310–9.

41. Allen J, Wojnarowska F. Linear IgA disease: the IgA and IgG response to dermal antigens demonstrates a chiefly IgA response to LAD285 and a dermal 180-kDa protein. Br J Dermatol 2003;149:1055–8.

42. Nishie W, Lamer S, Schlosser A, et al. Ectodomain shedding generates neoepitopes on collagen XVII, the major autoantigen for bullous pemphigoid. J Immunol 2010;185:4938–47.

43. Zillikens D, Herzele K, Georgi M, et al. Autoantibodies in a subgroup of patients with linear IgA disease react with the NC16A domain of BP1801. J Invest Dermatol 1999;113:947–53.

An Exception Within the Group of Autoimmune Blistering Diseases: Dermatitis Herpetiformis, the Gluten-Sensitive Dermopathy

Sarolta Kárpáti, MD, PhD, DrSc[a,b,*]

KEYWORDS

• Dermatitis herpetiformis • Gluten sensitivity • IgA precipitate
• Transglutaminase autoimmunity

Dermatitis herpetiformis (DH) is special among the classic autoimmune blistering skin diseases when considering its dermatologic symptoms, associated diseases, and pathomechanisms. The granular IgA precipitates present at the tips of the papillary dermis of the patients, an observation made by van der Meer in 1969 in Groningen,[1] proved to be pathognomonic for the disease. Contrary to other autoimmune blistering diseases, whereby tissue-bound and serum autoantibodies bind the same target molecule in the skin, no circulating IgA has been detected in DH sera reacting with normal tissue components of the sub-basal membrane zone or any other connective tissue particles within the healthy papillary dermis. The antigenicity of skin-bound IgA remained unknown for 3 decades, until 2002, when epidermal transglutaminase (TG3) was identified by the author's research group as its main antigen, an enzyme never detected in that area of the normal skin.[2] It has also been confirmed that DH patients have serum IgA autoantibodies to TG3. This article focuses on the clinical data concerning DH, rather than its detailed pathomechanism.

A version of this article was previously published in *Dermatologic Clinics 29:3*.

[a] Department of Dermatology, Venereology and Dermato-Oncology, Semmelweis University, Mária utca 41, Budapest 1085, Hungary; [b] Hungarian Academy of Sciences, Molecular Research Group, Mária utca 41, Budapest 1085, Hungary
* Corresponding author. Hungarian Academy of Sciences, Molecular Research Group, Mária utca 41, Budapest 1085, Hungary.
E-mail address: skarpati@t-online.hu

Immunol Allergy Clin N Am 32 (2012) 255–262
doi:10.1016/j.iac.2012.04.005
0889-8561/12/$ – see front matter © 2012 Elsevier Inc. All rights reserved.

SKIN SYMPTOMS AND DISEASE MANAGEMENT

DH can start at any age; rarely, it can be present in toddlers or in the very elderly, but the mean onset is generally in young adulthood or middle age. It is a chronic, very pruritic skin disease, characterized by 1- to 3-mm large papules, seropapules, vesicles, crusted erosions, and excoriations (**Fig. 1**). Rarely, larger blisters can also develop. The lesions heal with hypopigmentation or hyperpigmentation. In young patients, urticarial plaques might be the predominant skin symptoms (**Fig. 2**). The severe pruritus and scratching can result in extended lichenification (**Fig. 3**). In the majority of cases DH is a polymorphic skin disease, and only rarely presents as a bullous dermatosis.[3–5] Specific symptoms, not always present, are purpura on the fingers and toes, which alone may focus attention on the diagnosis (**Fig. 4**).

DH has a typical distribution of the skin symptoms; these are, in order of frequency (strongly supported by the author's personal observations): 1, elbows and knees; 2, buttock; 3, shoulders, middle line of the back, and scapula; 4, scalp; 5 (rarely), purpura on the fingers and toes (see **Figs 1–4**).[3,4]

Although severe DH is almost a continuous disease with some fluctuation in the severity and itch, it might also present as a relatively mild lichenification, with alternating

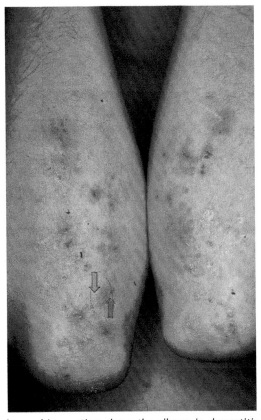

Fig. 1. Grouped polymorphic eruption above the elbows in dermatitis herpetiformis. Red arrow indicates the best site for a lesional biopsy for routine histology, and the blue arrow the best site for a perilesional biopsy for direct immunofluorescence.

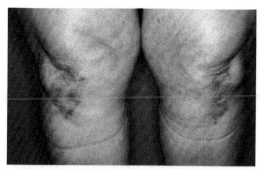

Fig. 2. Note the symmetric crusted erosions above the knees.

remissions and relapses: a few patients have skin disease only for a few days between long symptom-free periods. The symptom-free periods may only be in the warmer months when it is sunny. By contrast, in some DH patients sweating may induce disease progression in hot weather. There are patients who, without a gluten-free diet or other medication, remain free of skin symptoms for at least 6 months, in so-called spontaneous remission.[6] One must bear in mind that the underlying celiac disease (CD) and the possibility for further secondary disease development will persist. Spontaneous remissions are rare, but might develop and may last for years, life-long, or just for a short

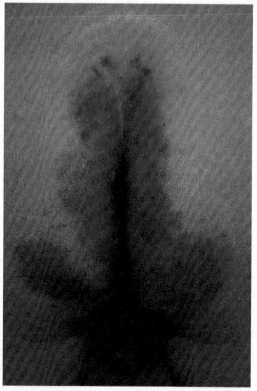

Fig. 3. Skin along the gluteal cleft is commonly involved in dermatitis herpetiformis: eczema-like chronic, livid erythema and mild lichenification without vesicles and crusts.

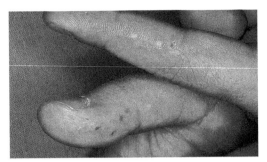

Fig. 4. Purpura on the fingers in dermatitis herpetiformis, a rare but specific sign.

time. Pruritus can precede the skin symptoms and rarely also challenge the otherwise symptom-free time of the patients.

Untreated DH can be a life-long disease with variable severity. Associated uncontrolled diabetes, autoimmune diseases, underlying tumors, and iodine challenges might induce permanent very severe skin symptoms. During pregnancy the disease may improve, but in some cases it is worse. The reason for iodine sensitivity of DH patients is unknown, but is common. A possible relationship with thyroid diseases also remains unraveled. The sensitivity can be proved by patch testing, but iodine-containing drugs also flare up the disease. One of the author's young patients underwent a thyrotoxic crisis together with a severe DH flare-up after one short visit to a salt cave suggested for her as a "natural therapy."

DIAGNOSIS CONFIRMATION

Diagnosis should be made by histologic and direct immunofluorescence (IF) analysis of the skin. The former sample should be taken from the lesional skin, the latter from perilesional, close to symptom-free tissue. On urticaria like lesions the presence of IgA, C3, and eventually IgM and IgG vasculitis is commonly associated with granular IgA and C3 staining of the dermis.[7] In the serum the presence of circulating IgA endomysial antibodies (EMA) or tissue transglutaminase (TG2) autoantibodies should be checked by indirect IF and by enzyme-linked immunosorbent assay (ELISA), respectively. The sensitivity and specificity of these tests are very high for CD, between or above 90% to 95%, whereas for DH it is less: about 75% to 90%. Serum samples from autoimmune diseases as well as sera from normal individuals treated by heat or pH shift might show nonspecific TG2 reactivity.[8,9] The TG3 antibodies (ELISA) are also gluten dependent and slowly disappear under gluten-free diet (GFD), but later than the EMA or TG2. TG3 antibodies are more commonly present in DH than in CD patients, and in DH patients they have higher avidity and affinity.[2,10,11] An upper gastroduodenoscopy and a small bowel histology is strongly advised to visualize and document the upper part of the gastroinstestine and to analyze the initial jejunal histology, due to its strong association with CD.[3,4]

Enteropathy and Malabsorption

The majority (75%–90%) of DH patients have an associated small bowel disease, a latent or silent CD. It persists and without treatment leads to malabsorption, which may induce secondary diseases: microcytic or macrocytic anemia due to iron, folate, or B12 deficiency, caries, alopecia due to zinc deficiency (see also dental problems), and early or very severe osteoporosis. Weight loss but also weight gain is possible, with unfavorable body mass index (BMI). Most patients have no typical gastrointestinal symptoms, but symptoms may include any of the following: diarrhea, constipation, bloating, abdominal discomfort or pain, and secondary lactose intolerance. Similarly to other gluten-sensitive enteropathy (GSE) patients, in DH patients with severe insulin-dependent diabetes, because of malabsorption the diabetes will be controlled only under a combined, strict GFD and diabetic diet. In childhood short stature, delayed development and puberty, or a high BMI might indicate the underlying GSE. Dental enamel defects, and mineralization disturbances of permanent and decidual teeth may be evident. Half of DH patients have celiac-type permanent-tooth enamel defects, milder than those described for severe celiac disease, and secondary severe caries or early tooth loss is also more common.[3–6,12,13] Although the skin can go into spontaneous remission,[3–6] the underlying CD and the possibility for further secondary disease development persist.

OTHER ASSOCIATED DISEASES
Autoimmune Diseases

Due to the high frequency of associated autoimmune diseases, the author recommends screening and following the patients for autoimmune thyroiditis, type 1 diabetes (anti-islet AB), lupus erythematosus, Sjögren syndrome, vitiligo, primary biliary cirrhosis, pernicious anemia, and alopecia areata.[14] Screening the family for DH, CD, and autoimmune diseases is suggested.

Neurologic Associations

Gluten sensitivity presenting with ataxia (gluten ataxia) is approximately one-quarter of the sporadic idiopathic cerebellar ataxia, the single most common cause of the disease.[15]

Rarely, gluten-induced axonal and demyelinating neuropathy, and myopathies have also been identified. In the central nervous system epilepsy, myoclonus, dementia, and multifocal leukoencephalopathy were detected in patients with GSE.[16]

Tumors

Long-lasting GSE is significantly more commonly associated with jejunal adenocarcinomas and lymphomas. Enteropathy-associated T-cell lymphomas encompass about 1% of the non-Hodgkin lymphomas, and these usually have a very poor prognosis. Other lymphomas, such as B or cutaneous lymphomas, have also been described. The relative risk of any lymphoma in untreated CD and DH is significantly enhanced, while a risk reduction is well documented under strict GFD.[17–19]

Other Disease Associations

Iodine sensitivity (cause is unknown), selective immunoglobulin A deficiency (more common also in CD), Down syndrome, and Turner syndrome have been reported.[3,4]

GENETIC BACKGROUND AND FAMILY SCREENING

There is no difference between CD and DH patients: HLA could be a nonspecific diagnostic marker for both diseases. Ninety-five percent of DH patients are HLA DQ2 positive with DQA1* 0501/DQB1*0201; DQA1*0501/DQB1*0202; DRB1*03/DRB1*05/07 alleles, while 5% of them are HLA-DQ8 positive and carry the DQA1*0301/DQB1*0302, DRB1*4 alleles.[6,20] Asiatic races lack this HLA pattern, therefore DH and CD are rare and in these patients because this association cannot be detected.

There are a few patients reported from Japan with only epidermal but not with tissue TG autoantibodies.[21]

GSE is more common among the family members of DH patients. Therefore it is strongly suggested to screen the first-degree and second-degree relatives for the presence of tissue TG antibodies (or EMA) to identify latent or silent forms of gluten sensitivity.[20]

TREATMENT

A strict, long-lasting (according to current knowledge life-long) GFD is the most advisable treatment for DH patients, which is healthy and seems to prevent the development of lymphomas and diseases associated with gluten-induced enteropathy and malabsoportion.[3–5] The GFD should be maintained in DH patients who become free from skin symptoms while on the diet. Also, patients with spontaneous regression need to take the diet because the GSE persists. The skin symptoms rarely disappear even under a strict GFD within a few weeks, and commonly persist for months or for a year. Gastroenterological and dietician consultations are necessary.

A secondary lactose intolerance might accompany the GSE, and in these cases a temporary lactose-gluten–free diet combination is advised.

In severe or insulin-resistant diabetic patients, only the combination of low-carbohydrate diet and GFD seems to be effective, because severe diabetes can be only stabilized if the enteropathy is reversed and the absorption is normalized. Low iodine intake like iodine-free salt, avoidance of fruit of meer (eg, shellfish), and GFD might be necessary for DH cases with iodine sensitivity. A dose of 50 to 150 mg dapsone per day could be a quick help for severe skin symptoms, because all DH patients react well to this medication. Dapsone, however, has no effect on the underlying GSE, nor on the secondary malabsorption and the enhanced risk of lymphomas. Dapsone may induce peripheral neuropathy and in glucose-6-phosphate–deficient patients, hemolysis. Rarely, it may be toxic to the bone marrow or might induce drug hypersensitivity syndrome. A high-dose vitamin C supplementation is suggested with dapsone to reduce methemoglobinemia.[12] In the first months of dapsone treatment blood counts, including reticulocyte counts, and bilirubin and liver enzyme values should be repeatedly determined. For more detailed information on dapsone, see the article elsewhere in this issue. Sunshine or ultraviolet A are beneficial for the skin symptoms and may keep mild cases in good condition, but cannot be considered as a sole treatment (personal observation by the author). In GFD refractory cases, patients should be screened for underlying diseases, particularly for tumors.[13]

DISEASE PATHOGENESIS: CLINICAL RELEVANCE

When and how the tolerance to alimentary gluten is lost in DH patients is not known exactly. The presence of IgA antibodies against gliadin and TG2 in the circulation prove the activity of enteropathy or a too short or improper diet adherence, therefore they should be regularly monitored. The major difference between CD and DH is the presence of skin symptoms, and the IgA precipitates in the papillary skin that may persist for years even in symptom-free patients. Furthermore, only in DH skin a pathologic epidermal TG3 is also deposited, colocalizing there with the granular IgA staining.[2,22,23] TG3-IgA immune complexes can be also detected in the small vessels of the papillary dermis.[7] These data show that DH can be considered as a gluten-induced immune-complex disease of the skin developing in some patients suffering from milder CD. The presence of cutaneous immune complexes also explains the purpura on the fingers and toes. The gluten-induced skin and small bowel pathology develops

Table 1 Dermatitis herpetiformis is a multidisciplinary disease: a guideline summary for patient care	
Skin	Skin histology (lesional) and direct IF for papillary IgA (perilesional)
Serum	Detect IgA to TG2 (ELISA) or endomysium (EMA, indirect IF), and TG3 (ELISA). Total serum IgA level
Gut	Gastroenterology consult: endoscopy/small bowel biopsy for H&E and IgA
Family	Screen the first- and second-degree relatives for gluten-sensitive diseases by IgA-TG2 antibody test (ELISA)
Associations	Autoimmune diseases, osteoporosis, enemal deficiencies, and neurologic symptoms. Correct the symptoms of malabsorption
Diet	Dietician consult; healthy, strict GFD; control the patients following the titer of serum IgA to TG2 or EMA. SLOW improvement! (months). Relapses indicate diet failure or tumor
Follow-up	Regular checkup for associated diseases. Be aware of the rare possibility of lymphoma development in patients under gluten-containing diet

Abbreviations: ELISA, enzyme-linked immunosorbent assay; EMA, endomysial antibodies; GFD, gluten-free diet; H&E, hematoxylin and eosin; IF, immunofluorescence; TG, transglutaminase.

only in genetically determined individuals who carry specific HLADQ8 or DQ2 haplotypes (see earlier discussion).

Although an interesting animal model of a gluten-sensitive skin disease was presented in HLA-DQ8 transgenic NOD mice, and this animal model demonstrated well the role of HLA molecules in gluten-induced immunologic reactions, a DH similar TG3 autoimmunity could not be reproduced.[24] It is likely that there are additional genetic or environmental factors that might contribute to gluten-dependent TG autoimmunity.[25,26]

MANAGEMENT OF DH

Management of DH will be discussed in more detail in the next issue, but a summary guideline is given in **Table 1**.

REFERENCES

1. van der Meer JB. Granular deposits of immunoglobulins in the skin of patients with dermatitis herpetiformis. An immunofluorescent study. Br J Dermatol 1969;81(7): 493–503.
2. Sárdy M, Kárpáti S, Merkl B, et al. Epidermal transglutaminase (TGase 3) is the autoantigen of dermatitis herpetiformis. J Exp Med 2002;195(6):747–57.
3. Collin P, Reunala T. Recognition and management of the cutaneous manifestations of celiac disease: a guide for dermatologists. Am J Clin Dermatol 2003; 4(1):13–20.
4. Kárpáti S. Dermatitis herpetiformis: close to unravelling a disease. J Dermatol Sci 2004;34(2):83–90.
5. Junkins-Hopkins JM. Dermatitis herpetiformis: pearls and pitfalls in diagnosis and management. J Am Acad Dermatol 2010;63(3):526–8.
6. Paek SY, Steinberg SM, Katz SI. Remission in dermatitis herpetiformis: a cohort study. Arch Dermatol 2011;147(3):301–5.
7. Preisz K, Sárdy M, Horváth A, et al. Immunoglobulin, complement and epidermal transglutaminase deposition in the cutaneous vessels in dermatitis herpetiformis. J Eur Acad Dermatol Venereol 2005;19(1):74–9.

8. Zöller-Utz IM, Esslinger B, Schulze-Krebs A, et al. Natural hidden autoantibodies to tissue transglutaminase cross-react with fibrinogen. J Clin Immunol 2010;30(2): 204–12.

9. Sárdy M, Csikós M, Geisen C, et al. Tissue transglutaminase ELISA positivity in autoimmune disease independent of gluten-sensitive disease. Clin Chim Acta 2007;376(1–2):126–35.

10. Marietta EV, Camilleri MJ, Castro LA, et al. Transglutaminase autoantibodies in dermatitis herpetiformis and celiac sprue. J Invest Dermatol 2008;128(2):332–5.

11. Dahlbom I, Korponay-Szabó IR, Kovács JB, et al. Prediction of clinical and mucosal severity of coeliac disease and dermatitis herpetiformis by quantification of IgA/IgG serum antibodies to tissue transglutaminase. J Pediatr Gastroenterol Nutr 2010;50(2):140–6.

12. Dunne J, Caron A, Menu P, et al. Ascorbate removes key precursors to oxidative damage by cell-free haemoglobin in vitro and in vivo. Biochem J 2006;399(3): 513–24.

13. Rubio-Tapia A, Murray JA. Classification and management of refractory coeliac disease. Gut 2010;59(4):547–57.

14. Neuhausen SL, Steele L, Ryan S, et al. Co-occurrence of celiac disease and other autoimmune diseases in celiacs and their first-degree relatives. J Autoimmun 2008;31(2):160–5.

15. Stamnaes J, Dorum S, Fleckenstein B, et al. Gluten T cell epitope targeting by TG3 and TG6; implications for dermatitis herpetiformis and gluten ataxia. Amino Acids 2010;39(5):1183–91.

16. Wills AJ, Turner B, Lock RJ, et al. Dermatitis herpetiformis and neurological dysfunction. J Neurol Neurosurg Psychiatry 2002;72(2):259–61.

17. Collin P, Pukkala E, Reunala T. Malignancy and survival in dermatitis herpetiformis: a comparison with coeliac disease. Gut 1996;38(4):528–30.

18. Viljamaa M, Kaukinen K, Pukkala E, et al. Malignancies and mortality in patients with coeliac disease and dermatitis herpetiformis: 30-year population-based study. Dig Liver Dis 2006;38(6):374–80.

19. Holmes GK, Prior P, Lane MR, et al. Malignancy in coeliac disease—effect of a gluten free diet. Gut 1989;30(3):333–8.

20. Karell K, Korponay-Szabo I, Szalai Z, et al. Genetic dissection between coeliac disease and dermatitis herpetiformis in sib pairs. Ann Hum Genet 2002;66(Pt 5–6):387.

21. Asano Y, Makino T, Ishida W, et al. Detection of antibodies against epidermal transglutaminase but not tissue transglutaminase in Japanese patients with Dermatitis herpetiformis. Br J Dermatol 2010. DOI: 10.1111/j.1365-2133.2010.

22. Dieterich W, Laag E, Bruckner-Tuderman L, et al. Antibodies to tissue transglutaminase as serologic markers in patients with dermatitis herpetiformis. J Invest Dermatol 1999;113(1):133–6.

23. Jaskowski TD, Hamblin T, Wilson AR. IgA anti-epidermal transglutaminase antibodies in dermatitis herpetiformis and pediatric celiac disease. J Invest Dermatol 2009;129(11):2728–30.

24. Marietta E, Black K, Camilleri M, et al. A new model for dermatitis herpetiformis that uses HLA-DQ8 transgenic NOD mice. J Clin Invest 2004;114(8):1090–7.

25. Koskinen LL, Korponay-Szabo IR, Viiri K, et al. Myosin IXB gene region and gluten intolerance: linkage to coeliac disease and a putative dermatitis herpetiformis association. J Med Genet 2008;45(4):222–7.

26. Blazsek A, Sillo P, Ishii N, et al. Searching for foreign antigens as possible triggering factors of autoimmunity: torque Teno virus DNA prevalence is elevated in sera of patients with bullous pemphigoid. Exp Dermatol 2008;17(5):446–54.

Pathophysiology of Dermatitis Herpetiformis: A Model for Cutaneous Manifestations of Gastrointestinal Inflammation

Adela Rambi G. Cardones, MD, Russell P. Hall III, MD*

KEYWORDS

• Dermatitis herpetiformis • Gastrointestinal inflammation
• Cutaneous autoimmune disease

Louis Duhring[1] proposed using the term dermatitis herpetiformis (DH) in 1884 to describe a cutaneous disease that was characterized by violent pruritus. Almost 1 century later, Cormane reported another key feature of this disease: the deposition of immunoglobulins at the dermoepidermal junction.[2] Shortly afterwards, it was described that 85% to 90% of patients with DH had granular and the rest linear, IgA deposits.[3,4] The third key feature was first described in 1966: these patients had an associated gastrointestinal disease, more specifically, a gluten-sensitive enteropathy (GSE).[5–7] Not only was it shown that this disease was GSE, but that dietary control was sufficient in abrogating the cutaneous symptoms of DH.[7,8] The association of GSE with DH was further correlated with the pattern of cutaneous IgA deposits by Lawley and colleagues,[9] who found that patients with clinical DH and an associated GSE had granular IgA deposits only in the skin. This finding defined the significance of DH as a model for an autoimmune disease that linked gastrointestinal mucosal immunity with cutaneous disease. Since that time, much has been done to describe the clinical and immunopathologic features of DH. Although the exact mechanism by which cutaneous lesions appear is still unclear, much has been uncovered in the pathophysiology of the disease.

A version of this article was previously published in *Dermatologic Clinics 29:3*.
Department of Dermatology, Duke University, DUMC 3135, Durham, NC 27710, USA
* Corresponding author. Room 4044, Purple Zone, Duke South, Durham NC, 27710-0001.
E-mail address: hall0009@mc.duke.edu

CLINICAL PRESENTATION

The classic cutaneous manifestations of DH, true to Duhring's original description, are markedly pruritic, symmetrically distributed papulovesicles that usually affect the extensor surfaces: scalp, especially the posterior hairline, elbows, knees, back, and buttocks.[1,10] Certainly variations exist, and frankly bullous, pustular, or eczematous lesions can sometimes be found. Patients can have only multiple erosions or small ulcerations, with or without crust, as a result of the severe pruritus. Rarely, atypical morphologies and locations, such as purpuric macules on the palms or tips of fingers,[11–13] can be found as presenting features, especially in children. The mucous membranes are only rarely, if ever, involved, but have certainly been reported as an initial manifestation of the disease.[14,15] The patients typically report a tingling or burning sensation 12 to 24 hours before the appearance of clinically evident lesions, which persists until the vesicle is broken and a crust is formed. DH typically presents in the second or third decade of life, with some investigators reporting a mean age of onset in the 40s, but it can certainly appear at any age.[16–19] The condition is chronic, but waxes and wanes with no clear triggering factors. This disease tends to be chronic, although around 12% of these patients can go into spontaneous remission.[20] Those who were 39 years or older at the age of onset and those who had already had longer duration of disease were more likely to experience remission. It is more prevalent among Anglo-Saxons and Scandinavians, with the estimated frequency between 10 and 39 per 100,000.[21,22] This frequency seems to be similar among Whites in the United States.[23] It is less common among other ethnic groups, such as African Americans and Asians, presumably because of differences in the frequency of HLA antigens associated with DH.[24–26] Furthermore, clinical variations may exist among different ethnicities. An increased incidence of fibrillar pattern of IgA deposits in the skin of patients with a clinical presentation consistent with DH has been reported in a Japanese cohort.[26] In addition, these Japanese patients seem to have a decreased frequency of GSE. It is not clear if this situation is because of a true difference in the pathogenesis of the disease, decreased exposure to gluten in the Japanese patients, or a less aggressive diagnostic approach to the potential gut disease. Although DH in the past has not been considered to be a familial disease, recent studies have indicated an indicated prevalence of both DH and isolated GSE in families. The incidence of familial occurrence (ie, a first-degree relative with DH) has been reported at 2.3% to 4.4%.[19,27,28] In a series from Finland, as many as 6.1% of patients with DH have first-degree relatives with celiac disease.[27]

HISTOLOGY AND IMMUNOPATHOLOGY

Histology of skin in DH is characterized by a subepidermal blister with a predominantly neutrophilic infiltrate in the dermal papillary tips,[18] although a mixed or even predominantly lymphocytic dermal infiltrate may also be found.[19,29] Direct immunofluorescence reveals granular deposition of IgA at the dermoepidermal junction in both involved and uninvolved skin as well as the oral mucosa.[30–32] However, IgA deposition is not evenly distributed in the skin of patients with DH.[33] Deposition is most intense in noninflamed perilesional skin, and is decreased in skin that has never been involved. Erythematous or lesional skin in patients with DH may not show IgA deposition, perhaps as a result of neutrophil destruction of the IgA. Therefore, the ideal site for a skin biopsy in DH is uninvolved, perilesional skin. Patients with isolated GSE without DH do not have cutaneous IgA deposition,[34] showing that this phenomenon is related to DH itself, and not the underlying GSE.

Complement deposition, specifically C3,[31,33,35,36] can be found along with IgA in the skin of patients with DH. There is evidence that IgA activates complement in DH via the alternative pathway.[35,37]

A fibrillar pattern of IgA deposition in a subset of patients with DH has also been described.[38–40] Although these patients typically have other clinical features consistent with DH, it has been suggested that these patients may have a higher incidence of atypical features, such as a urticarial or psoriasiform clinical presentation, the absence of GSE, or HLA-B8/DR3/DQ2 haplotype.[39] Some of these patients have been reported to lack circulating antibodies against tissue transglutaminase and endomysium.[40] Whether or not these patients represent a true distinct subset or variant of DH or another disease entity altogether remains to be seen.[41]

ASSOCIATED CONDITIONS

Patients with DH have an associated GSE. In contrast to patients with GSE alone, most patients with DH have little or no gastrointestinal symptoms, in spite of the almost invariable presence of demonstrable pathologic changes in the gastrointestinal tract when there is active cutaneous disease. Even when cutaneous disease is controlled with dapsone or sulfapyridine, the mucosal changes are persistent. Twenty percent to 30% of patients with DH have mild steatorrhea, and even fewer complain of bloating, diarrhea, and malabsorption. The gross and histologic changes of the small bowel in DH are identical, although less severe, to that found in isolated GSE or celiac disease. There is often patchy involvement, with changes confined to the small bowel, typically the jejenum. There is flattening of the intestinal villi, elongation of intestinal crypts, and flattening of the intestinal epithelial cells. A mononuclear infiltrate of plasma cells and lymphocytes is found in the lamina propria and intraepithelially. These changes persist even when cutaneous symptoms are controlled with dapsone and sulfapyridine but normalize with dietary therapy or strict avoidance of gluten.

Aside from GSE, several diseases are associated with DH. It has been reported that up to 41% of patients with DH have hypochlorhydria or achlorhydria, and most of these patients have gastric atrophy.[42] As many as 38% of patients with DH have been found to have thyroid microsomal antibodies, and patients with DH have a higher incidence of thyroid abnormalities, including hypothyroidism, thyroid nodules, and thyroid cancer.[43,44] Other autoimmune diseases have been reported to be associated with DH as well: systemic lupus erythematosus, dermatomyositis, myasthenia gravis, Sjögren syndrome, and rheumatoid arthritis.[45] IgA nephropathy has also been described in patients with DH, and mesangial changes and IgA deposition can be found even in the absence of overt renal symptoms.[46]

Patients with DH have been reported to have an increased risk of gastric lymphoma 2.3 times higher than the normal population, with the incidence as high as 6.4%.[47] However, others have reported a lower rate. Hervonen and colleagues[48] reported that only 1% of a series of 1104 patients with DH developed gastrointestinal lymphoma 2 to 31 years after the onset of DH and these patients were less likely to have adhered to adhere to a gluten-free diet. More recent reports have found no increased incidence of malignancy or mortality among patients with DH and matched controls.[49,50]

IMMUNOGENETICS

DH has striking HLA associations, specifically with class I antigens HLA-B8[51–53] and HLA-A1[54] and the class II antigens HLA-DR3 and HLA-DQw2.[54–56] Initial studies showed that 58% of patients with DH had HLA-B8, as opposed to 20% to 30% of normal controls. This same genetic marker was found to be present in 88% of patients with GSE as opposed to 22% of controls.[51–53,57] Furthermore, patients with GSE also have an increased frequency of HLA-A1, HLA-DR3 and HLA-DQw2, genetically linking DH and GSE. An even stronger association was found with HLA-DR3 and HLA-DQw2 because 95% and 100%, respectively, of patients with DH with confirmed granular IgA papillary dermal deposition expressed these markers.[55]

IMMUNOPATHOGENESIS

Although it is clear that gastrointestinal inflammation is integral in the pathophysiology of DH, the exact mechanism of antibody production as well as the cascade by which gastrointestinal inflammation translates into cutaneous disease is not known. Our laboratory has been interested in how the inflammatory response to gluten in patients with DH results in an itchy blistering skin disease with rare gastrointestinal symptoms, whereas patients with isolated GSE have no skin disease with significant gastrointestinal symptoms.

Patients with DH can control the appearance of cutaneous lesions by restricting themselves to a gluten-free diet. Moreover, eliminating gluten intake leads to a decrease and eventual clearance of IgA deposits in the skin.[58,59] Although the presence of IgA in the skin is well documented, we set out to determine if the IgA in the skin could be of gut origin. Evaluation of the IgA subclass present in DH skin revealed that the cutaneous IgA deposits were IgA1 and that joining chain could not be detected.[60] Because IgA1 is the predominant subclass of serum IgA whereas IgA2 is the predominant subclass in mucosal secretions this finding suggested that the IgA was not of mucosal origin. Patients with circulating IgA antibodies against reticulin and endomysium also had these antibodies in their intestinal secretions.[61] These studies showed that the presence of IgA autoantibodies in the serum is concordant with the presence of IgA antibodies in intestinal secretions. Furthermore, whereas normal gut secretions contained more IgA2, gut secretions from patients with DH were predominantly IgA1, showing that the IgA immune response in the gut was predominantly IgA1. Characterization of the serum and gastrointestinal IgA antibodies directed against dietary proteins revealed that both serum and intestinal antibodies had similar isoelectric spectrotypes and IgA subclass composition and that was distinct from the pattern seen with total serum IgA.[62] These studies showed that IgA1 antibodies in the serum can be of gut origin, linking closely the IgA immune response in the gut to the IgA deposits in DH skin. Although attempts to elute IgA from DH skin have not been successful, recent studies by Sardy and colleagues[63] and Donaldson and colleagues[64] have shown that the IgA in DH skin seems to bind to epidermal transglutaminase (eTG) in the dermis.

These studies, together with the clinical studies, have shown that the mucosal immune response to gluten can lead to IgA antibodies of mucosal origin, which can persist in circulation, and that a specific group of these antibodies, IgA antitransglutamase 3 (anti-TG3) (eTG), deposit in the skin. The mechanism of that binding remains unknown. However, these studies do not explain how the IgA deposits may relate to the development of skin lesions, nor do they explain the clinically different presentations of DH and isolated GSE.

eTG or TG3 has been identified as the target autoantigen in DH.[63,64] It is strongly expressed in the upper epidermis but may also be found in renal basement membrane. Patients with DH have detectable eTG in the papillary dermis, overlapping with the same sites that have IgA deposition. It was not found in sites where IgA was not found. It has been hypothesized that eTG is released from keratinocytes and drops to the basement membrane in response to trauma, and is subsequently bound by circulating IgA. Another hypothesis is that preformed circulating complexes of IgA and eTG deposit in the papillary dermis.[63] Evidence of the presence of these circulating complexes is shown by the precipitation of these complexes in vessel walls of patients with DH.[65] It has also been hypothesized that these dermal deposits are somehow the end product of a reaction against TG3 in kidneys. IgA nephropathy has been associated with DH, and mesangial deposits were detected in as many as 45% of patients with DH without any overt clinical signs of nephropathy.[46,66] Although IgA deposition in the kidney was not related to epidermal deposits or degree of gut involvement, this was associated with a high frequency of circulating IgA against gliadin and reticulin.[46] In 1 series of patients with DH, Jaskowski and colleagues[67] reported that serum eTG IgA compared with eTG IgA and IgG was more sensitive in detecting GSE; however, sensitivity of IgA anti-eTG was only 71%. Furthermore, dietary intake seems to correlate with eTG IgA; that is, avoidance of gluten resulted in the gradual decrease of antibody levels.

Despite the difference in the clinical presentations of patients with DH and those with isolated GSE, patients with DH and isolated GSE share many common features. In addition to sensitivity to gluten, patients with DH and those with isolated GSE share the same strong HLA association: HLA-A1, B8, DR3, DQ2.[68,69] Patients with DH and isolated GSE also both have circulating IgA anti-tissue and eTG antibodies and have the same typical histologic features of villous atrophy of the small intestine. In contrast most patients with DH do not complain of the bloating, abdominal cramps, and diarrhea that typically affect patients with isolated GSE. Only around 20% of patients with DH experience steatorrhea, and even fewer (<10%) have bloating, diarrhea, and malabsorption. In addition, patients with isolated GSE do not have cutaneous IgA deposits or skin blisters. These differences in clinical features may be because of a difference in the intestinal cytokine response to dietary gluten. Real-time polymerase chain reaction analysis of small bowel biopsies of patients with DH showed a greater expression of interleukin 4 (IL-4) mRNA and less expression of interferon γ (IFN-γ) compared with patients with isolated GSE.[70] In both DH and GSE, small bowel biopsy often shows a mononuclear infiltrate of plasma cells and lymphocytes if found in the lamina propria and intraepithelially. T-cell lines derived from small bowel mucosa of patients with DH were predominantly CD4+/IL-4+, and less frequently CD4+/IFN-γ+. In contrast, T-cell lines from isolated patients with GSE were predominantly CD8+ with a similar frequency of IL-4+ and IFN-γ+ cells.[71] In vitro culture of these T-cell lines with phorbol myristate acetate and ionomycin revealed that the T-cell lines produced IL-4 whereas isolated GSE T-cell lines produced both IL-4 and IFN-γ. These studies suggest that the increased expression of IL-4 mRNA in the gut of patients with DH when compared with patients with isolated GSE may modulate the inflammatory response and play a role in the lack of symptoms in patients with DH. T-cell receptor V_β expression also seems to be more restricted among patients with DH who continue to ingest gluten when compared with patients with isolated GSE on a gluten-containing diet.[72] Therefore, differences in the symptoms exhibited by patients with DH and isolated GSE may be the result of a difference in the local immune response and cytokine production.

Although these studies showed that patients with DH have an ongoing chronic mucosal immune response that results in mucosal IgA in the serum with deposition of IgA in the skin, the factors that lead to the development of the skin lesions were not clearly understood. Neutrophils play a central role in pathogenesis of the skin lesions seen in patients with DH. Histopathologic evaluation of involved skin shows neutrophil deposits in the papillary dermis. The development of skin lesions is also exquisitely responsive to dapsone, a drug known to inhibit neutrophil function, without changing the small bowel mucosal immune response. Patients with DH have a predominantly asymptomatic, chronic mucosal immune response in the gut, and control of the mucosal immune response through dietary gluten restriction can control the skin disease; it was certainly possible that the ongoing gut small bowel mucosa inflammation could partially prime both the skin and the circulating neutrophil with resultant skin blister formation. Evaluation of serum cytokine levels revealed that patients with DH with inactive skin disease secondary to use of dapsone but on a gluten-containing diet had increased levels of cytokines, including IL-8 and tumor necrosis factor α (TNF-α). We then compared the serum IL-8 and IgA anti-tissue trans-glutaminase levels in patients with DH before beginning a gluten-free diet and after an average of 24.5 months (range 0.5–40 months) of a gluten-free diet.[73] Patients who were placed on a gluten-free diet had a significant decrease in their serum IL-8 and IgA anti-tissue transglutaminase levels (**Fig. 1**). In contrast, those who were kept on a gluten-containing diet had persistently increased serum IL-8 and IgA anti-tissue transglutaminase levels even if their cutaneous disease was well controlled on dapsone or sulfapyridine. IL-8 mRNA message in small bowel biopsies of those on a gluten-containing diet was increased, whereas those patients on a gluten-free diet had IL-8 mRNA levels similar to normal controls. Thus, studies showed that the persistent mucosal immune response to gluten in the gut of patients with DH resulted in a chronic increase of proinflammatory cytokines in the circulation.

Neutrophils from patients with DH with active disease have an increased expression of CD11b when compared with those from patients with quiescent disease or normal controls. In addition, neutrophils from patients with DH with active disease had similar numbers of Fc IgA receptors but were able to bind more IgA compared with those from

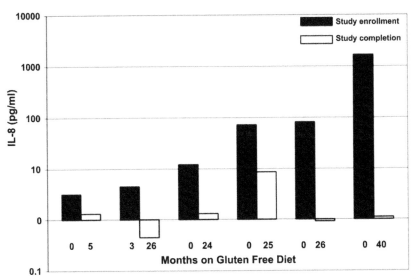

Fig. 1. Serum IL-8 levels in patients with DH on regular and gluten-free diets. Serum IL-8 is significantly reduced in patients with DH after maintaining a gluten-free diet (*open bars*) when compared with levels while on a gluten-containing normal diet (*solid bars*) (*P* = .0156, Wilcoxon signed rank test). (*From* Hall RP 3rd, Benbenisty KM, Mickle C, et al. Serum IL-8 in patients with dermatitis herpetiformis is produced in response to dietary gluten. J Invest Dermatol 2007;127:2159; with permission.)

normal controls.[74] This finding suggests that in patients with DH, the circulating neutrophils are partially primed to allow for increased adherence to endothelial cells and potentially responding to the cutaneous IgA deposits.

Although increased expression of CD11b is important in neutrophils exiting the circulation, the circulating neutrophil must also be able to firmly adhere to the cutaneous endothelium. Cytokines released from ongoing gastrointestinal inflammation may also be responsible for the activation of cutaneous endothelial cells. E-selectin is a type 1 protein that mediates stable arrest and adhesion of neutrophils on endothelial cells.[75,76] Normal inner arm skin in patients with DH on gluten-containing diets but without active skin lesions have an increased level of mRNA expression for E-selectin, when compared with E-selectin expression in the inner arm skin from normal individuals (**Fig. 2**).[77]

These studies show that in patients with DH on gluten-containing diets there is a chronic mucosal immune response that results in increases in circulating cytokines, including IL-8, a chemokine that is important in neutrophil function. This cytokine production is directly related to the mucosal immune response and is associated with increased expression of neutrophil CD11b and increased function of neutrophil Fc IgA receptors. This mucosal immune response is also associated with priming of the skin for an inflammatory response through a markedly increased expression of endothelial cell expression of E-selectin. However, the question remains why skin lesions are predominantly associated with the elbows, knees, buttocks, and other extensor areas. This regional localization may be caused by the constant minor trauma to extensor areas of the skin, and this trauma could result in local cytokine production in the skin, leading to chemotaxis of the partially primed neutrophils out of the blood vessels and into the skin at these sites of trauma. Minor trauma to the inner arm skin results in a striking increase in IL-8 and E-selectin mRNA and production of E-selectin protein in cutaneous endothelium.[78] This evidence supports the hypothesis that local trauma to the skin can establish the conditions necessary for neutrophils with an activated Fc IgA receptor to move into skin, localize to the dermal epidermal junction where the IgA deposits are found, and result in the development of blisters in the skin.

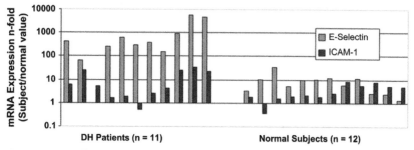

Fig. 2. Expression of E-selectin mRNA is increased in normal-appearing skin of patients with DH compared with normal individuals. mRNA expression represents fold expression of an individual compared with a constant single normal individual value. Expression of E-selectin mRNA in the skin of patients with DH is significantly increased compared with that seen in normal individuals (P = .0001, Mann-Whitney U test). No significant difference is seen in intercellular adhesion molecule 1 mRNA expression. (*From* Hall RP 3rd, Takeuchi F, Benbenisty KM, et al. Cutaneous endothelial cell activation in normal skin of patients with dermatitis herpetiformis associated with increased serum levels of IL-8, sE-Selectin and TNF-α. J Invest Dermatol 2006;126:1332; with permission.)

SUMMARY

DH is an autoimmune blistering skin disease in which antigen presentation in the gastrointestinal mucosa results in cutaneous IgA deposition and a distinct, neutrophil-driven cutaneous lesions. These studies taken in total provide us with a potential explanation of the pathophysiology of DH. The development of skin lesions in patients with DH is intimately linked to an active and chronic gastrointestinal mucosal inflammation as a result of persistent gluten challenge, resulting in a local immune response, with a production of mucosal IgA antibodies. This mucosal IgA reaches the circulation and a portion of it (potentially IgA anti-eTG) bind to skin. Because this IgA accumulates in the skin, the gastrointestinal mucosal immune response results in increased levels of circulating cytokines such as TNF-α and IL-8, which may partially prime neutrophils as well as activate cutaneous endothelial cells. Minor trauma to the skin increases local cytokine production, leading to egress of neutrophils and migration to the IgA at the dermal epidermal junction and the skin lesions of DH. This model is consistent with the clinical observation that skin disease can be prevented by use of dapsone, which affects neutrophil function but allows for ongoing gluten ingestion, or by a gluten-free diet, which inhibits the gut inflammation and controls the disease by stopping the inflammatory response in the gut. Our findings suggest that the qualitatively different immune response to gluten in the intestinal mucosa of patients with DH (increased IL-4 and decreased IFN-γ) results in minimal clinical symptoms, thus allowing the continued ingestion of gluten and the eventual development of the skin disease DH.

Although all of the elements of this hypothesis have not been firmly established they remain testable. Evaluation of patients for the induction of skin lesions by controlled trauma while on a gluten-containing diet would confirm the final pathway. In addition, further characterization of the mucosal immune response to gluten including antigen specificities and more defined cytokine patterns in patients with DH compared with isolated GSE is needed. This model suggests that chronic inflammation of an epithelial surface (lung, intestine, or skin), exposed to the external environment, whether by dietary or other environmental antigen, may have systemic effects through chronic cytokine expression or modulation of effector cells, which could play a critical role in disease processes in other organs. This model may provide a new way to understand the pathogenesis of other skin diseases associated with gastrointestinal inflammation such as pyoderma gangenosum or erythema nodosum, or explain association of seronegative inflammatory arthritis with inflammatory bowel disease.

REFERENCES

1. Duhring LA. Landmark article, Aug 30, 1884: dermatitis herpetiformis. By Louis A. Duhring. JAMA 1983;250(2):212–6.
2. Cormane RH. Immunofluorescence studies of the skin in lupus erythematosus and other diseases. Pathologica Eur 1967;2:170.
3. van der Meer JB. Granular deposits of immunoglobulins in the skin of patients with dermatitis herpetiformis. An immunofluorescent study. Br J Dermatol 1969; 81(7):493–503.
4. Chorzelski TP, Beutner EH, Jablonska S, et al. Immunofluorescence studies in the diagnosis of dermatitis herpetiformis and its differentiation from bullous pemphigoid. J Invest Dermatol 1971;56(5):373–80.
5. Marks J, Shuster S, Watson AJ. Small-bowel changes in dermatitis herpetiformis. Lancet 1966;2(7476):1280–2.

6. Shuster S, Watson AJ, Marks J. Coeliac syndrome in dermatitis herpetiformis. Lancet 1968;1(7552):1101–6.
7. Fry L, McMinn RM, Cowan JD, et al. Effect of gluten-free diet on dermatological, intestinal, and haematological manifestations of dermatitis herpetiformis. Lancet 1968;1(7542):557–61.
8. Fry L, McMinn RM, Cowan JD, et al. Gluten-free diet and reintroduction of gluten in dermatitis herpetiformis. Arch Dermatol 1969;100(2):129–35.
9. Lawley TJ, Strober W, Yaoita H, et al. Small intestinal biopsies and HLA types in dermatitis herpetiformis patients with granular and linear IgA skin deposits. J Invest Dermatol 1980;74(1):9–12.
10. Katz SI. Dermatitis herpetiformis. Clinical, histologic, therapeutic and laboratory clues. Int J Dermatol 1978;17(7):529–35.
11. Flann S, Degiovanni C, Derrick EK, et al. Two cases of palmar petechiae as a presentation of dermatitis herpetiformis. Clin Exp Dermatol 2010;35(2): 206–8.
12. Hofmann SC, Nashan D, Bruckner-Tuderman L. Petechiae on the fingertips as presenting symptom of dermatitis herpetiformis Duhring. J Eur Acad Dermatol Venereol 2009;23(6):732–3.
13. McGovern TW, Bennion SD. Palmar purpura: an atypical presentation of child-hood dermatitis herpetiformis. Pediatr Dermatol 1994;11(4):319–22.
14. Economopoulou P, Laskaris G. Dermatitis herpetiformis: oral lesions as an early manifestation. Oral Surg Oral Med Oral Pathol 1986;62(1):77–80.
15. Fraser NG, Kerr NW, Donald D. Oral lesions in dermatitis herpetiformis. Br J Dermatol 1973;89(5):439–50.
16. Gawkrodger DJ, Blackwell JN, Gilmour HM, et al. Dermatitis herpetiformis: diagnosis, diet and demography. Gut 1984;25(2):151–7.
17. Buckley DB, English J, Molloy W, et al. Dermatitis herpetiformis: a review of 119 cases. Clin Exp Dermatol 1983;8(5):477–87.
18. Rose C, Brocker EB, Zillikens D. Clinical, histological and immunopathological findings in 32 patients with dermatitis herpetiformis Duhring. J Dtsch Dermatol Ges 2010;8(4):265–70, 265–71.
19. Alonso-Llamazares J, Gibson LE, Rogers RS 3rd. Clinical, pathologic, and immunopathologic features of dermatitis herpetiformis: review of the Mayo Clinic experience. Int J Dermatol 2007;46(9):910–9.
20. Paek SY, Steinberg SM, Katz SI. Remission in dermatitis herpetiformis: a cohort study. Arch Dermatol 2011;147(3):301–5.
21. Moi H. Incidence and prevalence of dermatitis herpetiformis in a country in central Sweden, with comments on the course of the disease and IgA deposits as diagnostic criterion. Acta Derm Venereol 1984;64(2):144–50.
22. Reunala T, Lokki J. Dermatitis herpetiformis in Finland. Acta Derm Venereol 1978; 58(6):505–10.
23. Smith JB, Tulloch JE, Meyer LJ, et al. The incidence and prevalence of dermatitis herpetiformis in Utah. Arch Dermatol 1992;128(12):1608–10.
24. Hall RP, Clark RE, Ward FE. Dermatitis herpetiformis in two American blacks: HLA type and clinical characteristics. J Am Acad Dermatol 1990;22(3):436–9.
25. Hashimoto K, Miki Y, Nishioka K, et al. HLA antigens in dermatitis herpetiformis among Japanese. J Dermatol 1980;7(4):289–91.
26. Shibahara M, Nanko H, Shimizu M, et al. Dermatitis herpetiformis in Japan: an update. Dermatology 2002;204(1):37–42.
27. Reunala T. Incidence of familial dermatitis herpetiformis. Br J Dermatol 1996; 134(3):394–8.

28. Meyer LJ, Zone JJ. Familial incidence of dermatitis herpetiformis. J Am Acad Dermatol 1987;17(4):643–7.
29. Warren SJ, Cockerell CJ. Characterization of a subgroup of patients with dermatitis herpetiformis with nonclassical histologic features. Am J Dermatopathol 2002;24(4):305–8.
30. Seah PP, Fry L, Stewart JS, et al. Immunoglobulins in the skin in dermatitis herpetiformis and coeliac disease. Lancet 1972;1(7751):611–4.
31. Haffenden G, Wojnarowska F, Fry L. Comparison of immunoglobulin and complement deposition in multiple biopsies from the uninvolved skin in dermatitis herpetiformis. Br J Dermatol 1979;101(1):39–45.
32. Nisengard RJ, Chorzelski T, Maciejowska E, et al. Dermatitis herpetiformis: IgA deposits in gingiva, buccal mucosa, and skin. Oral Surg Oral Med Oral Pathol 1982;54(1):22–5.
33. Zone JJ, Meyer LJ, Petersen MJ. Deposition of granular IgA relative to clinical lesions in dermatitis herpetiformis. Arch Dermatol 1996;132(8):912–8.
34. Karlsson IJ, Dahl MG, Marks JM. Absence of cutaneous IgA in coeliac disease without dermatitis herpetiformis. Br J Dermatol 1978;99(6):621–5.
35. Provost TT, Tomasi TB Jr. Evidence for the activation of complement via the alternate pathway in skin diseases. II. Dermatitis herpetiformis. Clin Immunol Immunopathol 1974;3(2):178–86.
36. Katz SI, Hertz KC, Crawford PS, et al. Effect of sulfones on complement deposition in dermatitis herpetiformis and on complement-mediated guinea-pig reactions. J Invest Dermatol 1976;67(6):688–90.
37. Seah PP, Fry L, Mazaheri MR, et al. Alternate-pathway complement fixation by IgA in the skin in dermatitis herpetiformis. Lancet 1973;2(7822):175–7.
38. Kawana S, Segawa A. Confocal laser scanning microscopic and immunoelectron microscopic studies of the anatomical distribution of fibrillar IgA deposits in dermatitis herpetiformis. Arch Dermatol 1993;129(4):456–9.
39. Shimizu K, Hashimoto T, Fukuda T, et al. A Japanese case of the fibrillar type of dermatitis herpetiformis. Dermatology 1995;191(2):88–92.
40. Ko CJ, Colegio OR, Moss JE, et al. Fibrillar IgA deposition in dermatitis herpetiformis–an underreported pattern with potential clinical significance. J Cutan Pathol 2010;37(4):475–7.
41. Clements SE, Stefanato CM, Bhogal B, et al. Atypical dermatitis herpetiformis with fibrillar IgA deposition. Br J Dermatol 2007;157:17.
42. Gillberg R, Kastrup W, Mobacken H, et al. Gastric morphology and function in dermatitis herpetiformis and in coeliac disease. Scand J Gastroenterol 1985;20(2):133–40.
43. Gaspari AA, Huang CM, Davey RJ, et al. Prevalence of thyroid abnormalities in patients with dermatitis herpetiformis and in control subjects with HLA-B8/-DR3. Am J Med 1990;88(2):145–50.
44. Cunningham MJ, Zone JJ. Thyroid abnormalities in dermatitis herpetiformis. Prevalence of clinical thyroid disease and thyroid autoantibodies. Ann Intern Med 1985;102(2):194–6.
45. Reunala T, Collin P. Diseases associated with dermatitis herpetiformis. Br J Dermatol 1997;136(3):315–8.
46. Reunala T, Helin H, Pasternack A, et al. Renal involvement and circulating immune complexes in dermatitis herpetiformis. J Am Acad Dermatol 1983;9(2):219–23.
47. Leonard JN, Tucker WF, Fry JS, et al. Increased incidence of malignancy in dermatitis herpetiformis. Br Med J (Clin Res Ed) 1983;286(6358):16–8.

48. Hervonen K, Vornanen M, Kautiainen H, et al. Lymphoma in patients with dermatitis herpetiformis and their first-degree relatives. Br J Dermatol 2005;152(1): 82–6.
49. Lewis NR, Logan RF, Hubbard RB, et al. No increase in risk of fracture, malignancy or mortality in dermatitis herpetiformis: a cohort study. Aliment Pharmacol Ther 2008;27(11):1140–7.
50. Viljamaa M, Kaukinen K, Pukkala E, et al. Malignancies and mortality in patients with coeliac disease and dermatitis herpetiformis: 30-year population-based study. Dig Liver Dis 2006;38(6):374–80.
51. Katz SI, Hertz KC, Rogentine N, et al. HLA-B8 and dermatitis herpetiformis in patients with IgA deposits in skin. Arch Dermatol 1977;113(2):155–6.
52. White AG, Barnetson RS, Da Costa JA, et al. The incidence of HL-A antigens in dermatitis herpetiformis. Br J Dermatol 1973;89(2):133–6.
53. Katz SI, Falchuk ZM, Dahl MV, et al. HL-A8: a genetic link between dermatitis herpetiformis and gluten-sensitive enteropathy. J Clin Invest 1972;51(11): 2977–80.
54. Sachs JA, Awad J, McCloskey D, et al. Different HLA associated gene combinations contribute to susceptibility for coeliac disease and dermatitis herpetiformis. Gut 1986;27(5):515–20.
55. Hall RP, Sanders ME, Duquesnoy RJ, et al. Alterations in HLA-DP and HLA-DQ antigen frequency in patients with dermatitis herpetiformis. J Invest Dermatol 1989;93(4):501–5.
56. Karpati S, Kosnai I, Verkasalo M, et al. HLA antigens, jejunal morphology and associated diseases in children with dermatitis herpetiformis. Acta Paediatr Scand 1986;75(2):297–301.
57. Falchuk ZM, Rogentine GN, Strober W. Predominance of histocompatibility antigen HL-A8 in patients with gluten-sensitive enteropathy. J Clin Invest 1972; 51(6):1602–5.
58. Fry L, Leonard JN, Swain F, et al. Long term follow-up of dermatitis herpetiformis with and without dietary gluten withdrawal. Br J Dermatol 1982;107(6):631–40.
59. Leonard J, Haffenden G, Tucker W, et al. Gluten challenge in dermatitis herpetiformis. N Engl J Med 1983;308(14):816–9.
60. Hall RP, Lawley TJ, Heck JA, et al. IgA-containing circulating immune complexes in dermatitis herpetiformis, Henoch-Schonlein purpura, systemic lupus erythematosus and other diseases. Clin Exp Immunol 1980;40(3):431–7.
61. McCord ML, Hall RP 3rd. IgA antibodies against reticulin and endomysium in the serum and gastrointestinal secretions of patients with dermatitis herpetiformis. Dermatology 1994;189(Suppl 1):60–3.
62. Hall RP 3rd, McKenzie KD. Comparison of the intestinal and serum antibody response in patients with dermatitis herpetiformis. Clin Immunol Immunopathol 1992;62(1 Pt 1):33–41.
63. Sardy M, Karpati S, Merkl B, et al. Epidermal transglutaminase (TGase 3) is the autoantigen of dermatitis herpetiformis. J Exp Med 2002;195(6):747–57.
64. Donaldson MR, Zone JJ, Schmidt LA, et al. Epidermal transglutaminase deposits in perilesional and uninvolved skin in patients with dermatitis herpetiformis. J Invest Dermatol 2007;127(5):1268–71.
65. Preisz K, Sardy M, Horvath A, et al. Immunoglobulin, complement and epidermal transglutaminase deposition in the cutaneous vessels in dermatitis herpetiformis. J Eur Acad Dermatol Venereol 2005;19(1):74–9.
66. Helin H, Mustonen J, Reunala T, et al. IgA nephropathy associated with celiac disease and dermatitis herpetiformis. Arch Pathol Lab Med 1983;107(6):324–7.

67. Jaskowski TD, Hamblin T, Wilson AR, et al. IgA anti-epidermal transglutaminase antibodies in dermatitis herpetiformis and pediatric celiac disease. J Invest Dermatol 2009;129(11):2728–30.
68. Otley CC, Wenstrup RJ, Hall RP. DNA sequence analysis and restriction fragment length polymorphism (RFLP) typing of the HLA-DQw2 alleles associated with dermatitis herpetiformis. J Invest Dermatol 1991;97(2):318–22.
69. Fronek Z, Cheung MM, Hanbury AM, et al. Molecular analysis of HLA DP and DQ genes associated with dermatitis herpetiformis. J Invest Dermatol 1991;97(5): 799–802.
70. Smith AD, Bagheri B, Streilein RD, et al. Expression of interleukin-4 and interferon-gamma in the small bowel of patients with dermatitis herpetiformis and isolated gluten-sensitive enteropathy. Dig Dis Sci 1999;44(10):2124–32.
71. Hall RP 3rd, Smith AD, Streilein RD. Increased production of IL-4 by gut T-cell lines from patients with dermatitis herpetiformis compared to patients with isolated gluten-sensitive enteropathy. Dig Dis Sci 2000;45(10):2036–43.
72. Hall RP 3rd, Owen S, Smith A, et al. TCR Vbeta expression in the small bowel of patients with dermatitis herpetiformis and gluten sensitive enteropathy. Limited expression in dermatitis herpetiformis and treated asymptomatic gluten sensitive enteropathy. Exp Dermatol 2000;9(4):275–82.
73. Hall RP 3rd, Benbenisty KM, Mickle C, et al. Serum IL-8 in patients with dermatitis herpetiformis is produced in response to dietary gluten. J Invest Dermatol 2007; 127(9):2158–65.
74. Smith AD, Streilein RD, Hall RP 3rd. Neutrophil CD11b, L-selectin and Fc IgA receptors in patients with dermatitis herpetiformis. Br J Dermatol 2002;147(6): 1109–17.
75. Bevilacqua MP, Stengelin S, Gimbrone MA Jr, et al. Endothelial leukocyte adhesion molecule 1: an inducible receptor for neutrophils related to complement regulatory proteins and lectins. Science 1989;243(4895):1160–5.
76. Milstone DS, Fukumura D, Padgett RC, et al. Mice lacking E-selectin show normal numbers of rolling leukocytes but reduced leukocyte stable arrest on cytokine-activated microvascular endothelium. Microcirculation 1998;5(2–3):153–71.
77. Hall RP 3rd, Takeuchi F, Benbenisty KM, et al. Cutaneous endothelial cell activation in normal skin of patients with dermatitis herpetiformis associated with increased serum levels of IL-8, sE-Selectin, and TNF-alpha. J Invest Dermatol 2006;126(6):1331–7.
78. Takeuchi F, Sterilein RD, Hall RP 3rd. Increased E-selectin, IL-8 and IL-10 gene expression in human skin after minimal trauma. Exp Dermatol 2003;12(6):777–83.

Management of Dermatitis Herpetiformis

Adela Rambi G. Cardones, MD, Russell P. Hall III, MD*

KEYWORDS

• Dermatitis herpetiformis • Management
• Gluten-sensitive enteropathy • Pruritus

Dermatitis herpetiformis (DH) is a severely pruritic cutaneous disease characterized by markedly pruritic, symmetrically distributed papulovesicles that usually affect the extensor surfaces: the scalp (especially the posterior hairline), elbows, knees, back, and buttocks.[1,2] Histology of skin lesions in DH is characterized by a subepidermal blister with a predominantly neutrophilic infiltrate in the dermal papillary tips,[3] although a mixed or even predominantly lymphocytic dermal infiltrate may also be found.[4,5] Direct immunofluorescence reveals granular deposition of immunoglobulin A (IgA) at the dermal-epidermal junction in both involved and uninvolved skin as well as the oral mucosa.[6–10] Patients with DH have an associated gluten-sensitive enteropathy (GSE),[11] and dietary control is sufficient in abrogating the cutaneous symptoms of DH.[12,13] The condition is chronic, but it waxes and wanes with no clear triggering factors. This disease tends to be chronic, although approximately 10% to 12% of these patients can go into spontaneous remission.[14,15]

Epidermal transglutaminase (eTG) or transglutaminase 3 has been identified as the target autoantigen in DH.[16,17] Serum eTG IgA compared with tissue transglutaminase IgA and IgG was more sensitive in detecting GSE.[18] These serologic studies, however, should not be used to confirm the diagnosis of DH because the presence of IgA anti-eTG has a sensitivity for diagnosis of DH of only 70%. Furthermore, dietary intake seems to correlate with eTG IgA; that is, avoidance of gluten resulted in the gradual decrease of antibody levels.

TREATMENT

The 2 major options for the treatment of DH are medical treatment with dapsone or a sulfone drug and dietary treatment by the strict restriction of gluten intake.[19] Medical

---

A version of this article was previously published in *Dermatologic Clinics 29:4*.
Department of Dermatology, Duke University Medical Center, Durham, NC 27710, USA
* Corresponding author. Room 4044, Purple Zone, Duke South, 200 Trent Drive, Durham, NC 27710.
E-mail address: hall0009@mc.duke.edu

therapy with dapsone results in a rapid clinical improvement of skin findings, but it can be associated with side effects. Furthermore, it does not improve the gastrointestinal pathology in patients with DH.[20,21] On the other hand, dietary restriction of gluten has been proven to attenuate both the cutaneous and gastrointestinal signs and symptoms of DH.[13] However, this can be difficult because strict adherence is often required and the improvement of cutaneous symptoms may take weeks if not months.

Gluten-free Diet

Both the skin and the gastrointestinal manifestations of DH are gluten sensitive.[12,13] Leonard and coworkers[22] rechallenged 12 patients whose DH had previously been controlled on a gluten-free diet, and both the rash and the gastrointestinal changes recurred in response to the reintroduction of gluten. As many as 80% of patients with DH are able to stop or reduce their dose of dapsone on a strict gluten-free diet.[23] Those who are able to reduce but not completely eliminate gluten from their diet may see some benefit[15] but not enough to completely control their cutaneous symptoms.[20,24] Patients with DH treated with a gluten-free diet need at least 5 months before they are able to reduce their dapsone dose and anywhere from 8 to 48 months before they can stop dapsone treatment altogether.[12,13,23] In some patients, gluten restriction need not be lifelong because long-term remission can occur in as many as 10% to 12% of patients.[14,15] Bardella and colleagues[25] reported that 7 out of 38 patients who reverted to a normal, gluten-containing diet after an average of 8 years of gluten restriction continued to experience remission of their skin and gut disease after a mean follow-up of 12 years. Fry and coworkers[20] observed that macroscopic and microscopic small intestinal abnormalities among patients with DH on a gluten-free diet decreased significantly when compared with those who were on a normal diet, including a decrease in intraepithelial lymphocytic infiltration.[20] In this same study, they found that the improvement of cutaneous symptoms and gastrointestinal abnormality was directly related to the degree of strictness of the gluten-free diet. The incidence of lymphoma and other malignancies in patients with DH and GSE, although low, has been reported to increase when compared with the normal population.[26,27] Recent studies, however, have not found a similar increased risk of malignancy.[28] The reason for this discrepancy is not clear. It has been suggested that adherence to a gluten-free diet may play a role in moderating the risk of developing a malignancy, but a controlled study has not been done.[26,29] Van Der Meer and colleagues[30] have reported that an elemental diet can lead to the control of the eruption of DH. Kandunce and coworkers[31] have also shown that an elemental diet is effective at achieving control of DH often within 2 to 4 weeks.[31] Of interest, this effect seems to be independent of gluten ingestion. These studies suggest that other dietary proteins may also be important in the pathogenesis of dermatitis herpetiformis. IgA deposition in the skin appears to improve, albeit over a course of several years, on a gluten-free diet.[20,32,33] Fry and coworkers[32] noted that only 4 out of 23 patients with DH on a gluten-free diet had complete clearance of IgA deposition in their skin and only after several years. They further described that there was no difference in the quantity of IgA, as assessed by the amount of fluorescence, whether patients were controlled with a gluten-free diet alone, gluten-free diet and dapsone, dapsone alone, or in those in clinical remission. Frodin and coworkers[33] followed 32 patients with DH on either a gluten-free or gluten-reduced diet for 15 to 43 months and, although there was a decrease in the intensity of IgA deposition in the skin of these patients, none had a complete disappearance of cutaneous IgA deposition in spite of a good clinical response. In patients with DH controlled on a gluten-free diet and with clearance of cutaneous IgA deposition, gluten challenge results in the reappearance of cutaneous

IgA deposits within 1 month.[22] A more direct immunologic effect of a gluten-free diet is reflected in serum interleukin (IL)-8 levels among patients with DH. Serum IL-8 is elevated in patients with DH, and a gluten-free diet normalizes or reduces the amount of circulating IL-8 in these patients.[34] Patients with DH on a gluten-free diet had a decreased mRNA expression of IL-8 compared with those on a normal diet, suggesting that the elevated circulating IL-8 in patients with DH is produced in the intestinal mucosa as a response to gluten.[34]

Adherence to a gluten-free diet is effective in the majority of patients with DH at controlling the cutaneous manifestations of DH with a resultant decrease or elimination of the need for dapsone therapy. Even patients with DH with a normal initial small-bowel biopsy experience improvement of their rash when placed on a gluten-free diet.[35] In addition, a gluten-free diet may prevent or lessen the possibility of an increased risk of lymphoma and other malignancies in patients with DH. Adherence to a gluten-free diet, however, is difficult and requires significant knowledge and strong compliance by patients and their families. Fry and coworkers[20] noted that only 23 of 42 patients who thought that they were on a gluten-free diet were actually adhering to a strict gluten-free diet when evaluated by a dietitian. Consultation with a registered dietitian with expertise in gluten-free diets is often extremely valuable in improving patients' compliance with the diet. In addition, several patient groups are extremely useful for patients learning more about the diet (Celiac Sprue Association, csaceliacs.org).

Dapsone

The cutaneous signs and symptoms of DH can often be quickly and adequately controlled by 100 to 200 mg of dapsone with minimal side effects, although there is considerable variability in response.[19] Some patients require as little as 25 mg by mouth daily, whereas others may need up to 400 mg daily. Treatment can be initiated at a dosage of 100 mg daily unless patients have other significant risk factors, such as cardiovascular, pulmonary, or hematologic disease, and those who would likely not tolerate the hemolytic anemia and methemoglobinemia that may result from dapsone therapy. A complete review of the pharmacology and adverse effects of dapsone is beyond the scope of this review and readers are referred to several recent reviews for further information.[36,37] Most patients with DH will respond to dapsone within 24 to 36 hours of initiating the medication, and withdrawal of dapsone results in recurrence of signs and symptoms within 24 to 48 hours. Treatment with dapsone, however, does not alter gastrointestinal mucosal changes.[20,21] Furthermore, sulfone treatment does not appear to affect deposition of complement in the skin of patients with DH even when their cutaneous lesions were controlled.[38] This finding suggests that the therapeutic effect of dapsone is exerted at the effector cells of the cutaneous pathology; that is, there is neutrophilic infiltration of the skin and not at the initiation of the immunologic response, which is thought to occur when gut mucosa is exposed to gluten. Indeed, dapsone has been demonstrated to interfere with neutrophil chemotaxis[39] and the adhesion to antibodies[40] as well as with the release of IL-8 from keratinocytes.[41]

Careful monitoring of the side effects of dapsone is required. Aside from a careful history and physical examination to evaluate the cardiovascular, pulmonary, gastrointestinal, neurologic, and renal status of patients, a baseline complete blood count with differential, renal function test, liver function test, urinalysis, and G6PD level are recommended. Although a complete review of the pharmacology of dapsone is beyond the scope of the review, it is critical that the physician prescribing this drug be aware of the most severe adverse events. All patients will develop a dose-dependent hemolytic anemia with a resultant decrease in hemoglobin. In addition, some degree of methemoglobinemia will develop in all patients on dapsone, also in a dose-dependent manner. Concomitant administration of cimetidine, 400 mg by mouth 3 times a day, reduces dapsone-induced methemoglobinemia without affecting the clinical response in patients with DH.[42] Idiosyncratic side effects, including agranulocytosis, and hepatic function abnormalities may also occur. These side effects may be severe, and appropriate monitoring for side effects is essential. Because many of these side effects can be noted early and are reversible, monitoring of complete blood counts should be performed weekly for 1 month, every other week for 1 month, and then at 3- to 4-month intervals. Monitoring of liver and renal function should be performed periodically or as dictated by symptoms. Because many of these side effects are dose related, patients should be told not to adjust dapsone dosage without consulting their physician. Dapsone is also associated with a distal motor neuropathy. This event is relatively rare, but it is reversible and also requires monitoring by clinical examination and nerve-conduction studies as needed. Although dapsone is an extremely effective drug for the control of DH, the potential for toxicity is great and close follow-up is needed. Physicians who prescribe dapsone should be familiar with the pharmacology and adverse effects of the drug.[36,37] In addition, because of the unfamiliarity of some physicians with the use of dapsone, it is recommended that patients carry cards describing their use of dapsone and the associated adverse effects, including methemoglobinemia and a low-grade hemolytic anemia.

Sulfapyridine and Sulfasalazine

Sulfapyridine is an alternative medical treatment for DH, although less effective than dapsone, and patients are usually controlled with 1 to 2 g by mouth daily. This medication, however, is not readily available in the United States. Sulfasalazine, which is more readily available, is metabolized into 5-amino-salicylic acid (5-ASA) and sulfapyridine. Patients have been reported to respond to 2 to 4 g/d of sulfasalazine.[43,44] Once sulfasalazine is metabolized in the gut, most of the sulfapyridine is absorbed and excreted in the urine, whereas most of the 5-ASA remains in the gut and is thought to exert a local antiinflammatory effect that makes it useful in the treatment of inflammatory bowel disease.[45] It is not yet known if sulfasalazine exerts any effect on the gastrointestinal pathology in DH, but in one report of a patient with DH and ulcerative colitis, both the cutaneous and gastrointestinal symptoms improved on treatment with sulfasalazine.[46]

SUMMARY

The major treatment strategies for DH are gluten restriction or medical treatment with sulfones. Control of the cutaneous manifestations, but not the gastrointestinal changes, is rapid with dapsone. In addition to control of the cutaneous signs and symptoms of DH, dietary gluten restriction also induces improvement of gastrointestinal morphology and is possibly protective against the development of lymphoma.

REFERENCES

1. Duhring LA. Landmark article, Aug 30, 1884: dermatitis herpetiformis. By Louis A. Duhring. JAMA 1983;250(2):212–6.
2. Katz SI. Dermatitis herpetiformis. Clinical, histologic, therapeutic and laboratory clues. Int J Dermatol 1978;17(7):529–35.

3. Rose C, Brocker EB, Zillikens D. Clinical, histological and immunpathological findings in 32 patients with dermatitis herpetiformis Duhring. J Dtsch Dermatol Ges 2010;8(4):265–70, 265–71.
4. Alonso-Llamazares J, Gibson LE, Rogers RS 3rd. Clinical, pathologic, and immunopathologic features of dermatitis herpetiformis: review of the Mayo Clinic experience. Int J Dermatol 2007;46(9):910–9.
5. Warren SJ, Cockerell CJ. Characterization of a subgroup of patients with dermatitis herpetiformis with nonclassical histologic features. Am J Dermatopathol 2002;24(4):305–8.
6. Seah PP, Fry L, Stewart JS, et al. Immunoglobulins in the skin in dermatitis herpetiformis and coeliac disease. Lancet 1972;1(7751):611–4.
7. Haffenden G, Wojnarowska F, Fry L. Comparison of immunoglobulin and complement deposition in multiple biopsies from the uninvolved skin in dermatitis herpetiformis. Br J Dermatol 1979;101(1):39–45.
8. Nisengard RJ, Chorzelski T, Maciejowska E, et al. Dermatitis herpetiformis: IgA deposits in gingiva, buccal mucosa, and skin. Oral Surg Oral Med Oral Pathol 1982;54(1):22–5.
9. van der Meer JB. Granular deposits of immunoglobulins in the skin of patients with dermatitis herpetiformis. An immunofluorescent study. Br J Dermatol 1969; 81(7):493–503.
10. Chorzelski TP, Beutner EH, Jablonska S, et al. Immunofluorescence studies in the diagnosis of dermatitis herpetiformis and its differentiation from bullous pemphigoid. J Invest Dermatol 1971;56(5):373–80.
11. Marks J, Shuster S, Watson AJ. Small-bowel changes in dermatitis herpetiformis. Lancet 1966;2(7476):1280–2.
12. Fry L, McMinn RM, Cowan JD, et al. Gluten-free diet and reintroduction of gluten in dermatitis herpetiformis. Arch Dermatol 1969;100(2):129–35.
13. Fry L, McMinn RM, Cowan JD, et al. Effect of gluten-free diet on dermatological, intestinal, and haematological manifestations of dermatitis herpetiformis. Lancet 1968;1(7542):557–61.
14. Paek SY, Steinberg SM, Katz SI. Remission in dermatitis herpetiformis: a cohort study. Arch Dermatol 2011;147(3):301–5.
15. Garioch JJ, Lewis HM, Sargent SA, et al. 25 years' experience of a gluten-free diet in the treatment of dermatitis herpetiformis. Br J Dermatol 1994;131(4): 541–5.
16. Sardy M, Karpati S, Merkl B, et al. Epidermal transglutaminase (TGase 3) is the autoantigen of dermatitis herpetiformis. J Exp Med 2002;195(6):747–57.
17. Donaldson MR, Zone JJ, Schmidt LA, et al. Epidermal transglutaminase deposits in perilesional and uninvolved skin in patients with dermatitis herpetiformis. J Invest Dermatol 2007;127(5):1268–71.
18. Jaskowski TD, Hamblin T, Wilson AR, et al. IgA anti-epidermal transglutaminase antibodies in dermatitis herpetiformis and pediatric celiac disease. J Invest Dermatol 2009;129(11):2728–30.
19. Katz SI, Hall RP 3rd, Lawley TJ, et al. Dermatitis herpetiformis: the skin and the gut. Ann Intern Med 1980;93(6):857–74.
20. Fry L, Leonard JN, Swain F, et al. Long term follow-up of dermatitis herpetiformis with and without dietary gluten withdrawal. Br J Dermatol 1982;107(6):631–40.
21. Reunala T, Kosnai I, Karpati S, et al. Dermatitis herpetiformis: jejunal findings and skin response to gluten free diet. Arch Dis Child 1984;59(6):517–22.
22. Leonard J, Haffenden G, Tucker W, et al. Gluten challenge in dermatitis herpetiformis. N Engl J Med 1983;308(14):816–9.

23. Fry L, Seah PP, Riches DJ, et al. Clearance of skin lesions in dermatitis herpetiformis after gluten withdrawal. Lancet 1973;1(7798):288–91.

24. Ljunghall K, Tjernlund U. Dermatitis herpetiformis: effect of gluten-restricted and gluten-free diet on dapsone requirement and on IgA and C3 deposits in uninvolved skin. Acta Derm Venereol 1983;63(2):129–36.

25. Bardella MT, Fredella C, Trovato C, et al. Long-term remission in patients with dermatitis herpetiformis on a normal diet. Br J Dermatol 2003;149(5):968–71.

26. Hervonen K, Vornanen M, Kautiainen H, et al. Lymphoma in patients with dermatitis herpetiformis and their first-degree relatives. Br J Dermatol 2005;152(1):82–6.

27. Askling J, Linet M, Gridley G, et al. Cancer incidence in a population-based cohort of individuals hospitalized with celiac disease or dermatitis herpetiformis. Gastroenterology 2002;123(5):1428–35.

28. Lewis NR, Logan RF, Hubbard RB, et al. No increase in risk of fracture, malignancy or mortality in dermatitis herpetiformis: a cohort study. Aliment Pharmacol Ther 2008;27(11):1140–7.

29. Lewis HM, Renaula TL, Garioch JJ, et al. Protective effect of gluten-free diet against development of lymphoma in dermatitis herpetiformis. Br J Dermatol 1996;135(3):363–7.

30. van der Meer JB, Zeedijk N, Poen H, et al. Rapid improvement of dermatitis herpetiformis after elemental diet. Arch Dermatol Res 1981;271(4):455–9.

31. Kadunce DP, McMurry MP, Avots-Avotins A, et al. The effect of an elemental diet with and without gluten on disease activity in dermatitis herpetiformis. J Invest Dermatol 1991;97(2):175–82.

32. Fry L, Haffenden G, Wojnarowska F, et al. IgA and C3 complement in the uninvolved skin in dermatitis herpetiformis after gluten withdrawal. Br J Dermatol 1978;99(1):31–7.

33. Frodin T, Gotthard R, Hed J, et al. Gluten-free diet for dermatitis herpetiformis: the long-term effect on cutaneous, immunological and jejunal manifestations. Acta Derm Venereol 1981;61(5):405–11.

34. Hall RP 3rd, Benbenisty KM, Mickle C, et al. Serum IL-8 in patients with dermatitis herpetiformis is produced in response to dietary gluten. J Invest Dermatol 2007;127(9):2158–65.

35. Buckley DA, McDermott R, O'Donoghue D, et al. Should all patients with dermatitis herpetiformis follow a gluten-free diet? J Eur Acad Dermatol Venereol 1997;9(3):222–5.

36. Zhu YI, Stiller MJ. Dapsone and sulfones in dermatology: overview and update. J Am Acad Dermatol 2001;45(3):420–34.

37. Hall RP III, Mickle CP. Dapsone. In: Wolverton SE, editor. Comprehensive dermatologic drug therapy. Philadelphia: Saunders; 2001. p. 239–57.

38. Katz SI, Hertz KC, Crawford PS, et al. Effect of sulfones on complement deposition in dermatitis herpetiformis and on complement-mediated guinea-pig reactions. J Invest Dermatol 1976;67(6):688–90.

39. Wozel G, Blasum C, Winter C, et al. Dapsone hydroxylamine inhibits the LTB4-induced chemotaxis of polymorphonuclear leukocytes into human skin: results of a pilot study. Inflamm Res 1997;46(10):420–2.

40. Thuong-Nguyen V, Kadunce DP, Hendrix JD, et al. Inhibition of neutrophil adherence to antibody by dapsone: a possible therapeutic mechanism of dapsone in the treatment of IgA dermatoses. J Invest Dermatol 1993;100(4):349–55.

41. Schmidt E, Reimer S, Kruse N, et al. The IL-8 release from cultured human keratinocytes, mediated by antibodies to bullous pemphigoid autoantigen 180, is inhibited by dapsone. Clin Exp Immunol 2001;124(1):157–62.

42. Coleman MD, Rhodes LE, Scott AK, et al. The use of cimetidine to reduce dapsone-dependent methemoglobinemia in dermatitis-herpetiformis patients. Br J Clin Pharmacol 1992;34(3):244-9.
43. Goldstein BG, Smith JG Jr. Sulfasalazine in dermatitis herpetiformis. J Am Acad Dermatol 1990;22(4):697.
44. Willsteed E, Lee M, Wong LC, et al. Sulfasalazine and dermatitis herpetiformis. Australas J Dermatol 2005;46(2):101-3.
45. Klotz U. Clinical pharmacokinetics of sulphasalazine, its metabolites and other prodrugs of 5-aminosalicylic acid. Clin Pharmacokinet 1985;10(4):285-302.
46. Lambert D, Collet E, Foucher JL, et al. Dermatitis herpetiformis associated with ulcerative colitis. Clin Exp Dermatol 1991;16(6):458-9.

Corticosteroid Use in Autoimmune Blistering Diseases

John W. Frew, MBBS, MMed (Clin Epi)[a,b],
Dédée F. Murrell, MA, BMBCh, FAAD, MD, FACD[c],*

KEYWORDS

- Pemphigus • Pemphigoid • Linear IgA dermatosis
- Autoimmune blistering diseases • Corticosteroids

Corticosteroids have been used in the management of autoimmune blistering diseases (AIBD) for more than 50 years, and are an essential component in the pharmacologic management of these conditions. While providing rapid remission and ongoing control of the symptoms of AIBD, they come with a variety of potentially serious acute and long-term side effects. The advent of immunomodulating and immunosuppressive therapies has complemented the use of corticosteroids but have not usurped its pivotal role. The advent of evidence-based medicine (EBM) has reevaluated the various types of corticosteroids and forms of corticosteroid delivery in AIBD to ascertain whether any advantages of specific delivery systems or regimens exist. With rare diseases such as those that comprise AIBD, large randomized controlled trials are difficult to coordinate and accomplish, meaning a paucity of high-level evidence exists as to the best methods of corticosteroid use in these conditions. Experience and evidence from cross-discipline use of corticosteroids shows that careful monitoring of patients and simple preventive measures are effective in minimizing the adverse outcomes associated with their use. This article attempts to outline the current level of evidence for corticosteroid use in a variety of AIBDs, and discusses appropriate investigations and interventions to minimize or prevent the associated adverse effects.

PHARMACOLOGY OF CORTICOSTEROIDS

Corticosteroids are based around the cyclopentano-penanthrane nucleus, a conjoined series of three 6-carbon rings and one 5-carbon ring, a base structure shared by cholesterol and sex hormones.[1] All corticosteroids exhibit a double bond between

A version of this article was previously published in *Dermatologic Clinics 29:4.*
[a] St George Hospital, Kogarah, Sydney, NSW 2217, Australia; [b] Faculty of Medicine, University of Sydney, Sydney, NSW 2006, Australia; [c] Department of Dermatology, St George Hospital, University of New South Wales, Gray Street, Kogarah, Sydney, NSW 2217, Australia
* Corresponding author.
E-mail address: d.murrell@unsw.edu.au

Immunol Allergy Clin N Am 32 (2012) 283–294
doi:10.1016/j.iac.2012.04.008
0889-8561/12/$ – see front matter © 2012 Elsevier Inc. All rights reserved.

carbon atoms 4 and 5, as well as two ketone groups, attached to carbon atoms 3 and 20, which distinguish them from other cholesterol-based compounds. Different corticosteroids differ by their differing functional groups attached to the core ring structure as well as the oxidation state of the carbon atoms comprising the rings. General additions that increase corticosteroid potency include the insertion of a double bond between carbon atoms 1 and 2 (as in prednisone); the fluorination of carbon atoms 6 or 9 (as in clobetasol or dexamethasone); and the addition of a hydroxyl group at carbon atom 11 (as in clobetasol).[1]

Corticosteroids act through binding to glucocorticoid-specific receptors and altering transcription factors as well as diffusing through the cell membrane and acting directly on the cell nucleus.[2] Inflammatory inhibition is mainly achieved through the interaction with and inhibition of nuclear factor κB transcription factor, suppressing the production of chemokines and cytokines. Suppressed mediators include cyclooxygenases (COX), interleukins (IL) 1 through 6, tumor necrosis factor (TNF)-α, and macrophage colony stimulating factor. Although all of the exact mechanisms controlling the plethora of side effects of corticosteroids have not yet been elucidated, it is believed the majority of them are controlled through cyclic adenosine monophosphate–mediated pathways.[2] The end result is cytokine suppression, eosinopenia, lymphopenia, and monocytopenia. Neutrophilia is also observed. However, this is thought to be indirectly attributable to the decreased ability of neutrophils to migrate to the sites of inflammation due to cytokine suppression; neutrophil apoptosis is delayed as a result, contributing further to neutrophilia.[2]

Regarding the pharmacokinetics of corticosteroids, when prednisone is consumed orally it must be reduced enzymatically in the liver to prednisolone (the active product); this is done through reduction of a ketone group by the enzyme 11β-hydroxysteroidiesterase. Consequently, patients with hepatic dysfunction may have impaired conversion of prednisone to active prednisolone.[3] In these circumstances, administration of prednisolone would be more beneficial than prednisone in achieving the desired serum concentrations necessary for treatment. In patients with otherwise normal hepatic function, prednisone and prednisolone are drugs of equivalency. A table of steroid equivalencies for those drugs used in AIBDs is presented in **Table 1**.[1–4] With regard to conversion rates, serum concentrations for systemic steroids are roughly consistent. Measurements of equivalency for topical steroids have a much wider range than systemic steroids because, dependent on the site of measurement in the skin of the active ingredient, concentrations differ.[3] The measurements presented in **Table 1** are taken from studies wherein concentrations were measured in the dermis or at the dermoepidermal junction—the site of activity of disease and immune suppression. Consequently, concentrations in the epidermis would be much higher for topical steroids.

RESPONSIVENESS OF AIBD TO CORTICOSTEROIDS
Pemphigus Vulgaris/Pemphigus Foliaceus

Steroids have been used as the cornerstone of pemphigus management for more than 50 years.[5] The different types of corticosteroids used in pemphigus include oral prednisone/prednisolone as a continuous dosage for remission or maintenance therapy, and dexamethasone as used in oral pulsed dosage for remission and topical application for local or mucosal disease.[6] **Table 2** presents the current recommendations and levels of evidence available for corticosteroid use in AIBD. A recent systematic review and meta-analysis[5] examined a randomized controlled trial (RCT) of 22 participants comparing low-dose (45–60 mg/d) with high-dose (120–180 mg/d) oral prednisolone in a cohort of newly diagnosed pemphigus vulgaris (PV) and pemphigus foliaceus

Table 1
Equivalence table of different forms of corticosteroids used in AIBDs

Steroid Used	Converting To:					
	Prednisone/ Prednisolone[a]	Oral Dexamethasone	Intravenous Dexamethasone	Intravenous Hydrocortisone	Topical Betamethasone Valerate (0.1%)[b]	Topical Clobetasol Propionate (0.05%)[b]
Converting from: Prednisone/ prednisolone[a]	Multiply by 1 mg/kg/d	Multiply by 0.12 mg/kg/d	Multiply by 0.196 mg/kg/d	Multiply by 16 mg/kg/d	Multiply by 0.48 mg/kg/d	Multiply by 360 mg/kg/d
Oral dexamethasone	Divide by 0.12 mg/kg/d	Multiply by 1 mg/kg/d	Multiply by 0.61 mg/kg/d	Multiply by 133 mg/kg/d		
Intravenous dexamethasone	Divide by 0.196 mg/kg/d	Divide by 0.61 mg/kg/d	Multiply by 1 mg/kg/d			
Intravenous hydrocortisone	Divide by 16 mg/kg/d	Divide by 133.3 mg/kg/d		Multiply by 1 mg/kg/d		
Topical betamethasone valerate (0.1%)[b]	Divide by 0.48 mg/kg/d				Multiply by 1 mg/kg/d	
Topical clobetasol propionate (0.05%)[b]	Divide by 360 mg/kg/d					Multiply by 1 mg/kg/d

[a] Prednisone and prednisolone are assumed to be equivalent.
[b] Equivalence based on dermal concentrations.
Data from Refs.[1-4]

Table 2
Recommendations and level of evidence for corticosteroid use in autoimmune blistering diseases

Type of Corticosteroid	Recommendations and Level of Evidence				
	Pemphigus	Bullous Pemphigoid	Mucous Membrane Pemphigoid	Linear IgA Dermatoses	Epidermolysis Bullosa Acquisita
Prednisone/ prednisolone (oral)	A (2–3) Basic pillar of therapy. Optimal regimen (high dose vs low dose) unknown with current evidence	C (1) Can be used if topical unfeasible (evidence of deleterious effect compared with topicals in severe disease)	C (3)	I (3)	C (3) Associated with increased mortality and adverse effects
Dexamethasone (intravenous pulsed)	C (2–2) No evidence supporting its use over oral corticosteroids. Experts recommend use in recalcitrant disease	N/A	N/A	N/A	C (3) Use in intractable or severe disease
Dexamethasone (Mouthwash)	N/A	N/A	B (3)	N/A	N/A
Clobetasol propionate (0.05%)	C (3) Localized or mild disease	A (1) Recommended for severe disease over systemic corticosteroids based on 12-mo mortality rates	C (3)	I (3)	N/A
Betamethasone (topical)	C (3)	N/A	I (3)	I (3)	N/A

Key to Recommendations and Level of Evidence

Recommendations:

Level A: Good scientific evidence suggests that the benefits of the clinical service substantially outweigh the potential risks

Level B: At least fair scientific evidence suggests that the benefits of the clinical service outweigh the potential risks

Level C: At least fair scientific evidence suggests that there are benefits provided by the clinical service, but the balance between benefits and risks are too close for making general recommendations

Level D: At least fair scientific evidence suggests that the risks of the clinical service outweigh potential benefits

Level I: Scientific evidence is lacking, of poor quality, or conflicting, such that the risk-versus-benefit balance cannot be assessed

Levels of Evidence:

Level 1: Evidence obtained from at least one properly designed randomized controlled trial

Level 2-1: Evidence obtained from well-designed controlled trials without randomization

Level 2-2: Evidence obtained from well-designed cohort or case-control analytical studies, preferably from more than one center or research group

Level 2-3: Evidence obtained from multiple time series with or without the intervention. Dramatic results in uncontrolled trials might also be regarded as this type of evidence

Level 3: Opinions of respected authorities, based on clinical experience, descriptive studies, or reports of expert committees

Abbreviation: N/A, data not available.

(PF) patients.[7] Although the low number of participants made the study underpowered, no significant difference in the time to disease control was demonstrated.[7] All patients achieved remission in a time ranging from 5 to 42 days for the high-dose steroids and 7 to 42 days for the low-dose steroids. Rates of remission as recorded over a 5-year period were also not statistically significant ($P = .30$).[7]

Regarding pulsed corticosteroid use, an RCT of 22 participants[8] compared the efficacy of adjuvant pulsed oral dexamethasone (300 mg/d for 3 consecutive days, monthly) versus placebo in newly diagnosed patients concurrently treated with prednisolone and azathioprine. Although the small number of patients in the cohort contributed to the poor power of the study, no significant differences in the rates of remission or relapse were identified. Of importance, the rates of adverse outcomes or side effects were significantly higher among the pulsed-corticosteroid cohort when compared with the continuous-dosage cohort ($P<.01$).[8] It must be noted, however, that the patients enrolled in this particular study did not have severe or refractory disease, and that pulsed corticosteroids may have a useful role in those particular subgroups of patients.[6] At present no double-blinded placebo-controlled RCTs are available that evaluate pulsed corticosteroids in severe or refractory pemphigus, so the evidence supporting this stems from expert recommendation.[6] As the power of the study by Mentink and colleagues[8] was low, there is no evidence supporting the use of one intervention (dexamethasone or the control regimen) over the other. The study also commented that pulsed dexamethasone was associated with higher rates of corticosteroid-associated adverse effects.[8] These findings again highlight the importance of a dynamic corticosteroid regimen individualized for each patient depending on their individual disease severity, treatment response, and degree of adverse effects from therapy.

Topical corticosteroid use in PV and PF has been documented in several case reports,[9,10] and expert recommendations state that it may be useful in localized or mild disease.[6] No controlled trials exist to formally evaluate its efficacy, but strong corticosteroids such as betamethasone or clobetasol are typically used. For mucosal lesions, topical clobetasol propionate is typically used in mild disease, although mostly as an adjunct to systemic treatment.[6,11]

Bullous Pemphigoid

Corticosteroids, both oral and topical, are used widely in the management of bullous pemphigoid (BP), with topical preparations of high-potency steroids (such as clobetasol propionate) being used for mild to moderate disease and systemic corticosteroids used for more severe disease.[12] As BP is a disease of the elderly, mortality of those diagnosed with BP is relatively high, and despite the introduction of corticosteroids and other immunosuppressive and immunomodulating agents has not improved since the 1950s.[12,13] Debate is ongoing as to whether this is indicative of the underlying comorbidities inherent in the patient population and if the role of treatment actually improves mortality rates. Recent research by Parker and MacKelfresh[13] indicates that as the natural history of the disease is usually self limiting and the majority of patients succumb to causes unrelated to their BP, adverse effects primarily from systemic corticosteroids may actually increase the risk of mortality.[13]

A recent Cochrane systematic review and meta-analysis[12] examined an RCT of 26 participants comparing high-dose (1.25 mg/kg) and low-dose (0.75 mg/kg) oral prednisolone in patients with newly diagnosed BP.[14] Fifty-one percent of patients in the low-dose cohort patients achieved remission by day 21 compared with 64% of high-dose cohort patients. Power was limited by the small sample size of the study, and no significant difference between time to remission or overall mortality was revealed. A second study comparing oral prednisolone with methylprednisolone comprised 57 participants, monitored for 10 days. No significant difference in rates of remission or decrease in the number of bullous lesions was seen between the two treatment groups.[15] Self-reported pruritus scores were found to be significantly more improved in the methylprednisolone cohort than in the prednisolone cohort.[15] Examination of the methodology of the study shows that randomization and blinding were adequate, although the degree of allocation concealment is questionable, thus querying the reliability of this result.

The 2002 RCT by Joly and colleagues[16] comparing topical clobetasol propionate (0.05%) with oral prednisone demonstrated a significant advantage of topical clobetasol propionate (0.05%, 40 g/d) over oral prednisone (1 mg/kg/d) in individuals with severe BP (defined as more than 10 new blisters per day) in regard of overall mortality within 1 year of initiation of treatment. The significance of this finding increased when multiple regression analysis took into account age and functional status. Of importance, this study[16] also had adequate power to detect a decrease in the 1-year mortality rate in both severe and moderate disease groups. This result lends credence to the suggestion that in severe BP, systemic corticosteroids may have a deleterious effect on mortality rates when compared with topical high-potency corticosteroids. A follow-on study with 309 participants[17] found that lower doses of clobetasol propionate (0.05%, 10–30 g/d) had noninferior mortality rates than the standard regimen of 40 g/d in both severe and moderate disease. When adjusted for age and functional status, the investigators concluded that the lower doses were more beneficial to patients with both moderate and severe disease, with lower rates of mortality or life-threatening adverse effects (including sepsis and diabetes mellitus) than the original 2002 study.[12,17] Although the evidence may suggest that twice-daily topical corticosteroids more beneficial than oral dosing, the practicalities of application by elderly patients with multiple comorbidities is a significant barrier to the implementation of these recommendations.

Mucous Membrane Pemphigoid

Therapies for AIBD that involve mucous membranes are targeted at topical applications as well as the consideration of systemic corticosteroids in severe disease.

There is a paucity of evidence from RCTs regarding treatments for mucous membrane pemphigoid (MMP), cicatricial pemphigoid (CP), and other subtypes of AIBD that contain mucous membrane involvement. Expert recommendations cite topical therapies such as clobetasol propionate, betamethasone valerate, and dexamethasone mouthwashes.[18,19] A Cochrane review confirmed that the only RCT evidence related to MMP regarded the treatment of ocular involvement with dapsone or cyclophosphamide, dependent on disease severity.[19] There were no RCTs of steroid use in either MMP or epidermolysis bullosa acquisita (EBA). Furthermore, to date no reliable evidence sources (such as RCTs) have been found to further elucidate the efficacy of these topical treatments in these conditions.

Linear IgA Disease

Steroid use in linear IgA disease can be separated into topical and systemic regimens. While potent topical steroids such as clobetasol propionate 0.05% has been recommended for mild disease, it can also have a role in symptom control while the offending stimulant is removed in drug-induced disease.[20] No RCTs have been identified to date regarding the efficacy of corticosteroids in linear IgA disease, and expert recommendation quotes dapsone as a first-line agent,[20,21] with other immunosuppressive and immunomodulating agents such as mycophenolate mofetil (MMF) also having reports of successful treatment.[20] In this regard, systemic corticosteroids are only considered a useful adjunctive treatment in the setting of other therapies, and to this end evidence of its usefulness is lacking.

Epidermolysis Bullosa Acquisita

EBA is a recalcitrant AIBD in which treatment is known to be difficult. A recent Cochrane review found no RCTs of treatment modalities in EBA, although a handful of nonrandomized studies were found involving a wide variety of immunosuppressive and immunomodulating therapies.[22,23] Due to the adverse outcomes of the high-dose steroids needed to successfully control EBA, other management strategies such as intravenous immunoglobulins (IVIG) and anti-CD20 monoclonal antibodies (rituximab) have come to the fore as the mainstay of treatment in EBA.[22] While prednisone/prednisolone, 0.5 to 1.0 mg/kg/d is still included in the initial treatment regimen for EBA, recalcitrant or severe disease management concentrates on other immunomodulating therapies such as cyclosporine, plasmapheresis, and colchicine for maintenance therapy. Ishii and colleagues[23] state that pulsed corticosteroids may also be useful in severe disease, although these recommendations have not been borne out in randomized trials. Again, the rarity of the conditions comprising AIBD makes such evidence difficult to compile.

Pemphigoid Gestationis

Although there are no RCTs available assessing the effect of corticosteroids in this condition, as prednisone is relatively safe during the later stages of pregnancy and during breastfeeding as compared with many other systemic immunosuppressants, oral corticosteroids such as prednisone tend to be used.[24]

MINIMIZING THE ADVERSE EFFECTS OF CORTICOSTEROID USE

The side effects or adverse outcomes of corticosteroid use are both acute and chronic.

As outlined in **Table 3**, the adverse effects of corticosteroids range from weight gain and insulin resistance to acute psychopathology. Prevention strategies, ongoing management, and appropriate treatment of adverse effects that do arise are essential aspects of patient care in individuals with AIBD on systemic as well as widespread potent topical corticosteroids.[2] Evidence from studies in pemphigus have suggested that cumulative corticosteroid dose has a significant influence over the rate of adverse effects, again emphasizing the need for titration of steroid use according to individual patient responses.[2]

Metabolic Effects

The most common metabolic effects of corticosteroids include an increase of appetite and salt retention, leading to an increase in eating and drinking with consequent weight gain, hyperglycemia, and insulin resistance, along with hyperlipidemia. Baseline lipids (cholesterol, triglycerides, high-density lipoprotein, low-density lipoprotein, liver function tests) are advised prior to long-term glucocorticoids, with regular monitoring every 4 to 6 weeks, particularly when in combination with hepatotoxic drugs such as methotrexate.[2] Monitoring of weight and blood glucose should also be undertaken alongside lipids, especially in patients with preexisting diabetes or insulin resistance, as well as monitoring for hypertension. The effect of corticosteroids on blood glucose and lipids takes weeks to occur after starting therapy and a similar timeframe to return to normal after cessation of therapy.[2]

Table 3
Adverse outcomes from corticosteroid use in AIBDs and relevant strategies to prevent and alleviate effects

Adverse Effect	Timeframe of Onset	Prevention Strategies	Treatment Strategies
Weight gain	Weeks to months	Dose minimization	Dose minimization Diuretic therapy
Hyperglycemia/ insulin resistance	Weeks	Dose minimization	Endocrinology review Hypoglycemic therapy, insulin therapy
Osteoporosis	Years	Dose minimization Calcium and vitamin D supplementation Bisphosphonates	Calcium and vitamin D supplementation Bisphosphonates Acute management of fracture events
Osteonecrosis	Years	Dose minimization	
Myopathy	Weeks to years	Dose minimization Exercise, physiotherapy	Dose minimization Exercise, physiotherapy
Cataracts	Months	Dose minimization	Ophthalmology review Cataract removal
Glaucoma	Days to weeks	Dose minimization	Ophthalmology review
Psychopathology (Ranging from anxiety to acute psychosis)	Days-Weeks	Dose minimization	Neuropsychiatric review Antipsychotic medications
Hyperlipidemia	Weeks	Dose minimization Dietary modifications	Dietary modifications Statin therapy
Hypertension	Weeks	Dose minimization Dietary modifications (low sodium)	Dietary modifications (low sodium)
Infection/sepsis	Weeks	Dose minimization Prophylactic antibiotics Prophylactic antifungals Prophylactic antivirals	Acute medical management (intravenous antibiotics and supportive care)
Nausea/reflux	Days	Dose minimization Prophylactic proton pump inhibitors	Proton pump inhibitors Histamine-2 receptor antagonists

Data from Refs.[2,25–35]

Musculoskeletal Effects

One of the most common long-term effects of corticosteroid use is steroid-induced osteoporosis. With the greatest rate of bone mineral density loss occurring in the first 12 months of corticosteroid therapy, assessment and therapy before initiation of therapy or as soon as possible after initiation of therapy is vital.[25–27] Baseline bone mineral density (BMD) testing, along with serum calcium, magnesium, and vitamin D levels are necessary. The test considered most beneficial for BMD is dual x-ray absorption spectrometry (DEXA), due to a combination of its low radiation levels and reproducibility.[25,26] Yearly BMD testing along with ensuring adequate supplementation of calcium (recommended 1500 mg/d) and vitamin D (recommended 800 IU/d) can help minimize osteoporosis.[25,26] Other prophylactic pharmacologic therapies include bisphosphonates such as alendronate and risendronate.[27,28] Rheumatologic guidelines recommend administration of bisphosphonates to all men and postmeno-pausal women on long-term corticosteroid therapy of greater than 5 mg prednisone per day.[26] Nonpharmacologic methods aimed at maintaining bone mineral density in the setting of long-term corticosteroid use include a low sodium diet (to help prevent calcium loss from the renal tubules) and minimizing caffeine and alcohol intake.[25,26] Muscle atrophy and weakness is a delayed complication of systemic steroids, with little that can be done to prevent it; gentle exercise can help to keep the muscles as strong as possible.

Neuropsychiatric Effects

Central nervous system effects of high-dose corticosteroids can include disturbing psychiatric symptoms, which can have rapid onset of several days after initiation of therapy. Affective disturbances including depression and hypomania can be seen at moderate doses, but psychosis and mania are almost exclusively seen at doses above 20 mg/d.[29] One retrospective analysis in patients with multiple sclerosis taking steroids was able to identify individuals at risk by previous episodes of major depres-sion prior to the onset of disease.[29] Factor analysis in a cohort of systemic lupus eryth-ematosus (SLE) patients on systemic glucocorticoids showed that hypoalbuminemia was a significant predisposing factor to corticosteroid-induced psychosis in that patient population.[30] Insomnia is a common complaint present at low doses, and in elderly populations cognitive impairment, particularly memory loss, may manifest.[31] While preventive measures encompass monitoring and education as well as appro-priate dosing regimens, treatment of psychosis with various antipsychotic medica-tions has been documented as effective.[30]

Cardiovascular Effects

The risk of ischemic heart disease and cardiac failure is increased in individuals on long-term corticosteroid therapy greater than 7.5 mg of prednisone per day, as per the result of a case-control study of more than 50,000 individuals.[32] The risk as measured by odds ratios was greater for current users of systemic glucocorticoids than for previous users. Although the risk was not as great for cerebrovascular disease as with cardiovascular disease, the results have not been verified in RCTs and, hence, general recommendations on prevention or monitoring of patients on systemic corti-costeroids are currently inappropriate.

Gastrointestinal Effects

Corticosteroids have been reported to be associated with an increased risk of peptic ulcer disease, gastritis, and gastroesophageal reflux disease. Several studies have quantified the increased risk as marginally significant for glucocorticoids alone, although in combination with nonsteroidal anti-inflammatory drugs (NSAIDs), a signif-icant elevation in the risk for gastroenterological complications above the level attrib-utable to NSAIDs alone is detectable within the first 3 months of use.[33] Current expert recommendations in other fields do not recommend prophylaxis with proton pump inhibitors (PPIs) in the setting of glucocorticoids alone, but it can be considered for those individuals taking both glucocorticoids and NSAIDs.[33] It is the authors' practice, and that of other dermatologists in the field, to prescribe PPIs to AIBD patients on chronic, high-dose corticosteroids. No information is available as to the effect of COX-2–specific NSAIDs combined with systemic corticosteroids.

Ophthalmologic Effects

Posterior subcapsular cataracts are a well-documented adverse effect of prolonged corticosteroid use. These bilateral, slowly developing cataracts can usually be distinguished clinically from senile cataracts. Findings from rheumatologic research suggests that younger patients, particularly children, are more susceptible to the formation of cataracts, and that doses equivalent to less than 10 mg prednisolone per day can still cause significant increases in the rates of cataract formation when compared with matched controls.[34] Anecdotally, several of the authors' pemphigus patients have had to undergo cataract surgery. Increased intraocular pressure can also occur within months of systemic corticosteroid use, mimicking open-angle glaucoma, although it is much more commonly a risk with ocular use of corticosteroids.[2] Patients with preexisting glaucoma have an increased sensitivity to corticosteroids and risk of disease progression, and regular ophthalmologic reviews are a necessary part of monitoring side effects in these patients.[35]

Risk of Infection

The risk for potentially serious infection in AIBD patients, particularly those on long-term corticosteroid therapy combined with other immunosuppressive therapy, is high. Expert recommendations suggest the consideration of prophylaxis for *Candida* and/or *Pneumocystis* infections in patients with high-dose MMP.[2] Although no clear consensus guidelines are available concerning infectious prophylaxis in AIBD, Williams and Nesbitt[2] state that trimethoprim-sulfamethoxazole or dapsone are acceptable options for bacterial prophylaxis, with dapsone having additional anti-inflammatory properties. Valacyclovir can be used for viral prophylaxis for herpes simplex, and chlorhexidine/miconazole mouthwashes are appropriate for oral candidiasis prophylaxis.[2] Concerns over tuberculosis reactivation with individuals on immunosuppressive regimens have led rheumatologic authorities to suggest baseline chest radiographs and tuberculin skin testing prior to long-term immunosuppressive therapies. Opinions vary as to the appropriateness of these investigations in those on glucocorticoids alone, as most concern centers around the use of TNF-α inhibitors, such as infliximab and rituximab.[2] Drugs such as rituximab are being used as first-line treatment for pemphigus patients who have significant contraindications to high-dose corticosteroids.[16] Cost-benefit analyses in the short term may find that oral corticosteroids are cheaper than topical alternatives and biological therapies, but the longer term costs of the sequelae of high-dose steroids, listed above, have yet to be properly evaluated.

EXPERT RECOMMENDATIONS

Corticosteroids are a central tenet in the management of AIBD, and it is unlikely that any ethics committee would permit RCTs of placebos versus systemic steroids in the acute phases of these diseases, because the mortality decreased so dramatically when steroids were introduced for pemphigus. The focus is to minimize side effects with the lowest doses of corticosteroids or an alternative mode of application that is possible for efficacy.

REFERENCES

1. Bikowski J, Pillai R, Shroot B. The position not the presence of the halogen in corticosteroids influences potency and side effects. J Drugs Dermatol 2006; 5(2):125–30.

2. Williams LC, Nesbitt LT Jr. Update on systemic glucocorticosteroids in dermatology. Dermatol Clin 2001;19(1):63–77.
3. McClain R, Yentzer B, Fledman S. Comparison of skin concentration following topical versus oral corticosteroid treatment: reconsidering the treatment of common inflammatory dermatoses. J Drugs Dermatol 2009;8(12):1076–9.
4. Tóth G, Westerlaken B, Eilders M, et al. Dexamethasone pharmacokinetics after high-dose oral therapy for pemphigus. Ann Pharmacother 2002;36:1109.
5. Martin L, Agero AL, Werth V, et al. Interventions for pemphigus vulgaris and pemphigus foliaceus [review]. Cochrane Database Syst Rev 2009;1:CD006263.
6. Harman KE, Albert S, Black MM. Guidelines for the management of pemphigus vulgaris. Br J Dermatol 2003;149:926–37.
7. Ratnam K, Phay K, Tan C. Pemphigus therapy with oral prednisolone regimens: a five year study. Int J Dermatol 1990;29:363–7.
8. Mentink L, Mackenzie M, Toth G, et al. Randomized control trial of adjuvant oral dexamethasone pulse therapy in pemphigus vulgaris. Arch Dermatol 2007;143: 570–6.
9. Lapiere K, Caers S, Lambert J. A case of long standing pemphigus vulgaris on the scalp. Dermatology 2004;209:162–3.
10. Baykal C, Azizlerli G, Thoma-Uszynski S, et al. Pemphigus vulgaris localized to the nose and cheeks. J Am Acad Dermatol 2002;47:875–8.
11. Dagistan S, Goregen M, Miloglu O, et al. Oral pemphigus vulgaris: a case report with review of the literature. J Oral Sci 2008;50(3):359–62.
12. Kirtschig G, Middleton P, Bennett C. Interventions for bullous pemphigoid. Cochrane Database Syst Rev 2010;10:CD002292.
13. Parker S, MacKelfresh J. Autoimmune blistering diseases in the elderly. Clin Dermatol 2011;29(1):69–79.
14. Morel P, Guillaume JC. Treatment of bullous pemphigoid with prednisolone only: 0.75 mg/kg/day versus 1.25 mg/kg/day. A multicenter randomized study. Ann Dermatol Venereol 1984;111(10):925–8 [in French].
15. Dreno B, Sassolas B, Lacour P, et al. Methylprednisolone versus prednisolone methylsulfobenzoate in pemphigoid: a comparative multicenter study. Ann Dermatol Venereol 1993;120:518–21 [in French].
16. Joly P, Roujeau JC, Benichou J, et al. A comparison of oral and topical corticosteroids in patients with bullous pemphigoid. N Engl J Med 2002;346(5):321–7.
17. Joly P, Roujeau JC, Benichou J, et al. A comparison of two regimens of topical corticosteroids in the treatment of patients with bullous pemphigoid: a multicenter randomized study. J Invest Dermatol 2009;129(7):1681–7.
18. Knudson RM, Kalaaj AN, Bruce AJ. The management of mucous membrane pemphigoid and pemphigus. Dermatol Ther 2010;23(3):268–80. Available at: http://onlinelibrary.wiley.com/doi/10.1111/dth.2010.23.issue-3/issuetoc.
19. Kirtschig G, Murrell D, Wojnarowska F, et al. Interventions for mucous membrane pemphigoid and epidermolysis bullosa acquisita. Cochrane Database Syst Rev 2003;1:CD004056.
20. Korman N. Linear IgA bullous dermatosis. In: Lebwohl M, Heymann W, Berth-Jones J, et al, editors. Treatment of skin disease. Comprehensive therapeutic strategies. 2nd edition. London: Mosby Elsevier Ltd; 2006. p. 358–60.
21. Shimizu S, Natsuga K, Shinkuma S, et al. Localized linear IgA/IgG bullous dermatosis. Acta Derm Venereol 2010;90:621–4.
22. Kirtschig G, Murrell DF, Wojnarowska F, et al. Interventions for mucous membrane pemphigoid and epidermolysis bullosa acquisita. Cochrane Database Syst Rev 2000;4:CD004056.

23. Ishii N, Takahiro Hamada T, Dainichi T, et al. Epidermolysis bullosa acquisita: What's new? J Dermatol 2010;37:220–30.
24. Jenkins RE, Hern S, Black MM. Clinical features and management of 87 patients with pemphigoid gestationis. Clin Exp Dermatol 1999;24(4):255–9.
25. Gulko PS, Mulloy AL. Glucocorticoid-induced osteoporosis: pathogenesis, prevention and treatment. Clin Exp Rheumatol 1996;14:199–206.
26. American College of Rheumatology Ad Hoc Committee on Glucocorticoid-Induced Osteoporosis recommendations for the prevention and treatment of glucocorticoid induced osteoporosis. Arthritis Rheum 2001;44(7):1496–503.
27. Stoch SA, Saag KG, Greenwald M, et al. Once-weekly oral alendronate 70 mg in patients with glucocorticoid induced bone loss: a 12 month randomizes, placebo controlled clinical trial. J Rheumatol 2009;36(8):1705–14.
28. Cohen S, Levy R, Keller M, et al. Risendronate therapy prevents corticosteroid induced bone loss: a twelve month, multicenter, randomized, double blind placebo controlled parallel group study. Arthritis Rheum 1999;42(11):2309–18.
29. Minden S, Orav J, Schildkraut J. Hypomanic reactions to ACTH and prednisone in treatment for multiple sclerosis. Neurology 1988;38(10):1631–4.
30. Chau SY, Mok CC. Factors predictive of corticosteroid psychosis in patients with systemic lupus erythematosus. Neurology 2003;61(1):104–7.
31. Keenan P, Jacobson M, Soleymani R, et al. The effect on memory of chronic prednisone treatment in patients with systemic disease. Neurology 1996;47(6): 1396–402.
32. Souverein P, Berars A, Van Staa T. Use of oral glucocorticoids and risk of cardiovascular and cerebrovascular disease in a population based case-control study. Heart 2004;90(8):859–65.
33. Gabriel S, Jaakkimainen L, Bombardier C. Risk for serious gastrointestinal complications related to use of non steroidal anti inflammatory drugs, a meta analysis. Ann Intern Med 1991;115(10):787–96.
34. McDougall R, Sibley J, Haga M, et al. Outcome in patients with rheumatoid arthritis receiving prednisone compared to matched controls. J Rheumatol 1994;21(7):1207–13.
35. Trikudanathan S, McMahon GT. Optimum management of glucocorticoid treated patients. Nat Rev Endocrinol 2008;4:62–71.

Azathioprine in the Treatment of Autoimmune Blistering Diseases

Volker Meyer, MD, Stefan Beissert, MD*

KEYWORDS
- Azathioprine • Autoimmune blistering diseases • Pemphigus
- Bullous pemphigoid

HISTORY OF AZATHIOPRINE

The pharmaceutical precursor of azathioprine was originally 6-mercaptopurine. 6-Mercaptopurine was synthesized in 1951 by GB Elion and GH Hitchings using techniques reported by Fisher and Traube.[1] 6-Mercaptopurine was first used in 1953 in children with acute lymphatic leukemia.[2] Later, Calne,[3] a young surgeon who later became professor of surgery at Cambridge, successfully treated dogs after renal transplantation with 6-mercaptopurine in 1960, but because of the high toxic potential of the drug it was not found suitable for long-term treatment of humans with solid-organ transplants. Subsequently, it was shown that one of the derivatives of 6-mercaptopurine found by Elion and Hitchings, BW 57-322, presented with less bone marrow toxicity[4] but was as immunosuppressive as 6-mercaptopurine. To protect 6-mercaptopurine from being rapidly metabolized, an imidazole ring had been biochemically connected via the sulfur atom at position 6 of 6-mercaptopurine and thereby azathioprine was finally developed (**Fig. 1**). The first successful allogeneic renal transplant using a combination of azathioprine and corticosteroids was initiated in 1963.[5] Azathioprine is now used in particular for the treatment of autoimmune diseases, such as autoimmune blistering diseases, inflammatory bowel disease, multiple sclerosis, and lupus, to name a few.

STRUCTURE AND METABOLISM

About 88% of azathioprine is ingested and 12% excreted via the gut.[6] Nearly all the incorporated azathioprine is metabolized because only 2% is being excreted

---

A version of this article was previously published in *Dermatologic Clinics 29:4*.

The authors declare no conflict of interest.

Department of Dermatology, University of Muenster, Von-Esmarch-Str. 58, D-48149 Muenster, Germany

* Corresponding author.

E-mail address: beisser@uni-muenster.de

doi:10.1016/j.iac.2012.04.009
0889-8561/12/$ – see front matter © 2012 Elsevier Inc. All rights reserved.
immunology.theclinics.com

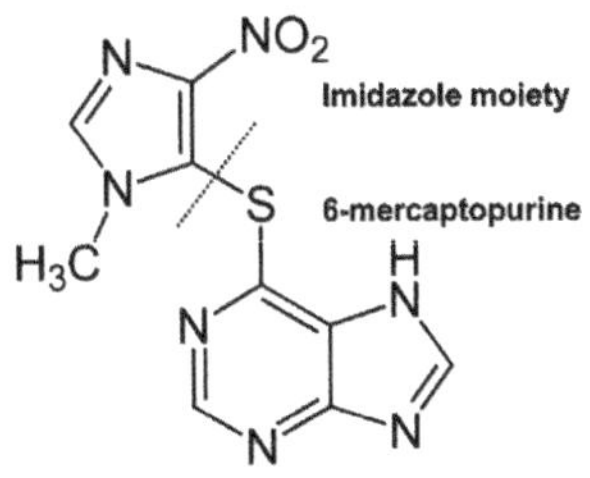

NO₂

Imidazole moiety

6-mercaptopurine

H₃C

Fig. 1. Structure of azathioprine. The dashed line marks the cleavage site.

unchanged in the urine. The highest serum levels can be found approximately 2 hours after oral application and the half-life is approximately 5 hours. After uptake, azathioprine is nonenzymatically cleaved into its imidazole derivatives (methylnitroimidazole moiety) and 6-mercaptopurine (see **Fig. 1**). Three enzymes have been reported to compete for the cleavage of azathioprine (**Fig. 2**).[7] Thiopurine S-methyltransferase (TPMT) is able to catabolize 6-mercaptopurine into the nontoxic 6-methyl mercaptopurine. Xanthine oxidase (XO) produces the nontoxic inactive metabolite 6-thiouric acid. A lack in one of these enzymes, XO and TPMT, leads to an increased production of toxic metabolites via the hypoxanthine phosphoribosyltransferase (HPRT) pathway. A lack of TPMT activity is normally caused by genetic mutations, whereas XO might be blocked by XO inhibitory drugs such as allopurinol, which is one of the most commonly prescribed drugs in Europe and North America. The enzyme HPRT metabolizes 6-mercaptopurine into 6-thioinosine 5-monophosphate (6-TIMP). This product is processed by TPMT to active methylated metabolites or is phosphorylated to 6-thioinosine triphosphate (6-TITP). 6-TITP is converted to 6-TIMP by inosine triphosphate pyrophosphohydrolase (ITPA). A lack of ITPA, often seen in Asian populations,[8] leads to an increase in the level of toxic 6-TITP and induces corresponding side effects, such as leukopenia, gastrointestinal disturbances, or elevated liver function test results (for details concerning side effects see later discussion).

6-TIMP is converted by inosine monophosphate dehydrogenase and guanosine monophosphate synthetase into the principal active 6-thioguanine nucleotides. These nucleotides are converted by TPMT into inactive methylated metabolites.

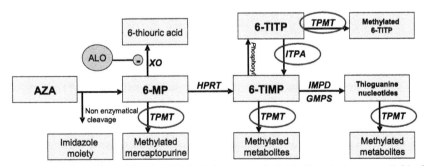

Fig. 2. Metabolism of azathioprine. Encircled enzymes indicate that tests are available for these enzymes for assessment of azathioprine's potential toxicity. ALO, allopurinol; AZA, azathioprine; GMPS, guanosine monophosphate synthetase; HPRT, hypoxanthine phosphoribosyltransferase; IMPD, inosine monophosphate dehydrogenase; ITPA, inosine triphosphate pyrophosphohydrolase; 6-MP, 6-mercaptopurine; 6-TIMP, 6-thioinosine monophosphatase; 6-TITP, 6-thioinosine triphosphatase; TPMT, thiopurine S-methyltransferase; XO, xanthine oxidase.

In patients with Lesch-Nyhan syndrome, reduced expression of HPRT can be detected, which makes these patients less suitable for azathioprine treatment. Although most of the therapeutic effects of azathioprine are dependent on the HPRT pathway, there is experimental evidence that the imidazole derivatives of azathioprine might also be effective.[9]

AZATHIOPRINE IN BULLOUS PEMPHIGOID

In 1971, Greaves and colleagues[10] introduced azathioprine into the treatment of bullous pemphigoid. Before that, most patients had been treated with systemic corticosteroid monotherapy to prevent recurrent blister formation. It was reported by Greaves and colleagues[10] that in 8 of 10 patients with bullous pemphigoid, no prednisone mainte-nance therapy was needed for preventing relapses, whereas azathioprine was given at a dose of 2.5 mg/kg body weight per day.

In a small prospective clinical trial in 1978, Burton and colleagues[11] examined azathi-oprine (2.5 mg/kg/d, n = 12) plus prednisone (30–80 mg/d) versus prednisone alone (n = 13). No significant difference between both groups was found concerning the over-all disease control. The prednisone-sparing effect was statistically significant. In the azathioprine group, a cumulative average dose of 3688 mg of prednisone was used for more than 3 years, whereas 6732 mg was used in the prednisone monogroup for the same period. In 1993, Guillaume and colleagues[12] found no significant difference in disease control between prednisone monotherapy (1 mg/kg/d, n = 31) and azathio-prine (100–150 mg/d, n = 36) plus prednisone therapy. However, the prednisone-sparing effect has not been investigated in this study.

In a national randomized trial in 2007, Beissert and colleagues[13] compared treat-ment with methylprednisolone (0.5 mg/kg/d) with either azathioprine (2 mg/kg/d, n = 38) or mycophenolate mofetil (1 g twice a day, n = 35). The results showed no significant differences in the primary outcome (ie, complete healing of skin lesions) and a tendency to faster healing in the azathioprine group (azathioprine 23.8 ± 18.9 days vs mycophenolate mofetil 42.0 ± 55.9 days, P value is nonsignificant). Moreover, similar corticosteroid doses were used to control disease. Mycophenolate mofetil was significantly less liver toxic compared with azathioprine, which can be an advantage especially in elderly patients.

A Cochrane review concluded from the available study results that the addition of azathioprine in the treatment of bullous pemphigoid had not been established.[14] The results of several studies concerning the treatment of bullous pemphigoid with azathioprine are summarized in **Table 1**.

AZATHIOPRINE IN PEMPHIGUS

The treatment of pemphigus vulgaris and pemphigus foliaceus usually does not differ significantly. Most investigators did not specify in their reports whether patients with pemphigus foliaceus or vulgaris had been treated.

The use of azathioprine for the treatment of pemphigus was introduced in 1969, when Krakowski and colleagues[15] presented the first case report of a woman with pemphigus-vulgaris treated successfully with azathioprine. At the same time, Aberer and colleagues[16] published a case series of 4 patients describing the use of azathioprine as "steroid saving and beneficial" in patients with pemphigus. In 1977, Lever and Schaumburg-Lever[17] pub-lished a retrospective analysis of 63 patients with pemphigus. The investigators treated patients (n = 12) with prednisone monotherapy and the other patients in this cohort (n = 51) with a combination of azathioprine, cyclophosphamide, or methotrexate and prednisone. In this report, azathioprine was described as "steroid saving and effective."

Table 1
Use of azathioprine in bullous pemphigoid (case reports are not included)

Investigators	Year	N	AZA Dose	Main Outcome
Greaves et al[10]	1971	10	2.5 mg/kg/d	8/10 symptom free, no prednisone needed
van Dijk & van Velde[44]	1973	5	75–250 mg/d	4/5 excellent response
Burton & Greaves[45]	1974	12	2.5 mg/kg/d	12/12 excellent response
Ahmed et al[46]	1977	15	1.5 mg/kg/d	Reduces duration of maintenance, steroid sparing
Burton et al[11]	1978	12	2.5 mg/kg/d	Steroid sparing, but control of disease not significantly different from steroid alone
Guillaume et al[12]	1993	36	100–150 mg/d	No significant difference to steroid monotherapy concerning disease control
Beissert et al[13]	2007	73	2 mg/kg/d	No significant differences in primary outcome between AZA + MP and MMF + MP, tendency of faster healing in AZA-treated patients

Abbreviations: AZA, azathioprine; MMF, mycophenolate mofetil; MP, methylprednisolone; N, number of patients treated with azathioprine.

The investigators' therapeutic approach is still known as Lever's regime. Initially, patients receive a high dose of prednisone (up to 2 mg/kg body weight) in combination with azathioprine 2.0 to 2.5 mg/kg. After cessation of new blister formation and reepithelization of erosions, the prednisone dose is reduced to 40 mg/d, while the azathioprine dose remains unchanged. Further proceedings depend on the individual's clinical development. Normally, the prednisone dose is gradually reduced over a period of several months.

There are only a few prospective randomized trials reported on pemphigus. Beissert and colleagues[18] examined 38 patients with pemphigus vulgaris or pemphigus foliaceus and found no significant differences between treatment with azathioprine and mycophenolate mofetil, both in combination with methylprednisolone, concerning remission of disease and corticosteroid-sparing effects. The patients treated with azathioprine received a median methylprednisolone dose of 8.916 ± 29.844 mg. In the mycophenolate mofetil–treated group, patients received a median of 9.334 ± 13.280 mg methylprednisolone (n = nonsignificant). The mean duration of follow-up was 438 days in both groups. However, the time needed to achieve disease control in 50% of the patients was about 30 days in the azathioprine group compared with 75 days in the mycophenolate mofetil group. Perhaps the inhibition of at least 3 enzymatic pathways by azathioprine (see **Fig. 2**) is able to induce a faster response in comparison with mycophenolate mofetil, which inhibits primarily 1 signaling pathway. Nevertheless, after 200 days of treatment, the patients in the mycophenolate mofetil group had a remission rate of 90%, whereas those who were treated with azathioprine had a remission rate of 75%. After 600 days, this trend persisted because 20% of patients with pemphigus were still not achieving effective control with azathioprine compared with 10% of patients using mycophenolate. The recurrence rate was similar in both groups.

In another study with 120 patients analyzed, Chams-Davatchi and colleagues[19] found no significant difference concerning disease remission between azathioprine and mycophenolate mofetil, but the patients treated with azathioprine showed significantly less steroid consumption. These findings indicate that azathioprine is well suited for first-line treatment of pemphigus. Rose and colleagues[20] compared dexamethasone-cyclophosphamide pulse therapy with oral methylprednisolone/azathioprine therapy in pemphigus. A tendency was found in favor of methylprednisolone/azathioprine concerning complete remissions.

In IgA pemphigus, azathioprine showed no considerable effect. Dapsone is usually the first-line treatment.[21] For pemphigus vegetans, azathioprine seems to work in individual cases.[22] For treatment of refractory patients, disease control has been reported under the corticosteroid/azathioprine regimen using additionally photopheresis or retinoids.[23,24]

In paraneoplastic pemphigus, therapy for the underlying malignancy is essential. Concomitant treatment with azathioprine and other immunomodulatory drugs has been reported, but it is difficult to conclude whether any of them will reliably affect the prognosis of the disease because its mortality approaches 90%.[25] Lam and colleagues[26] presented a case of a 77-year-old man with chronic conjunctivitis, acanthosis nigricans, and pemphigus-like mucocutaneous lesions. Further examinations revealed an underlying bronchogenic squamous cell carcinoma (SCC). Although skin lesions resolved with oral prednisone and azathioprine (100 mg/d) therapy, the conjunctivitis and mucous membrane erosions persisted. Verrini and colleagues[27] described another patient with paraneoplastic pemphigus who showed good response to azathioprine (100 mg/d) but died after a short time after initiation of treatment.

The importance of systemic corticosteroids in the treatment of pemphigus is clearly documented. Because the reports show a tendency in favor of azathioprine concerning corticosteroid-sparing effects and no significant differences regarding disease control, the authors suggest using azathioprine as first-line therapy in mild to moderate cases of pemphigus. Mycophenolate mofetil seems to be a valid second-line choice. In severe and rapidly progressing cases, dexamethasone/cyclophosphamide pulse therapy should be considered.

Because pemphigus is a chronic disease, long-term follow-up studies (>3 years) are clearly needed. A Cochrane review concluded from the available study results that the optimal immunomodulatory agent in the treatment of pemphigus has not yet been found. Although azathioprine and cyclophosphamide did show advantages concerning the steroid-sparing effect, mycophenolate showed superior disease control.[28]

The results of several studies concerning the treatment of pemphigus with azathioprine are shown in **Table 2**.

AZATHIOPRINE IN OTHER AUTOIMMUNE BLISTERING DISEASES

Several case reports show that azathioprine can be effective in cicatricial pemphigoid. These reports demonstrate that azathioprine is able to control disease and prevent progression. However, azathioprine showed no beneficial effect on already existing scars and cicatrizing vegetation. Unfortunately, there are no randomized or blinded trials available. The results of relevant case reports concerning the treatment of cicatricial pemphigoid are shown in **Table 3**.

Pemphigus can also develop in children, which is a rare event in Europe and North America. Some reports center around therapy for juvenile pemphigus with azathioprine and demonstrate the efficiency of azathioprine in children with pemphigus.[29] The results of important case reports concerning the use of azathioprine in juvenile pemphigus are shown in **Table 4**.

AZATHIOPRINE DURING PREGNANCY

The use of immunomodulatory agents during pregnancy should always be extremely well considered. Azathioprine is able to cross the human placenta.[30] The fetal liver

Table 2
Use of azathioprine in pemphigus (most case reports are not included)

Investigators	Year	N	AZA Dose	Main Outcome
Krakowski et al[15]	1969	1	75–150 mg	Control of disease after 4 mo
Aberer et al[16]	1969	4	1–3 mg/kg/d	Steroid saving and beneficial
Burton et al[47]	1970	4	2.5 mg/kg/d	3 of 4 with excellent response, but relapse after discontinuation of AZA; 1 patient dropped out because of severe side effects
Roenigk & Deodhar[48]	1973	10	50–250 mg/d	7, excellent; 2, good; 1, fair
van Dijk & van Velde[44]	1973	5	50–200 mg/d	5/5 excellent response
Lever & Schaumburg-Lever[17]	1977	6	50–150 mg/d	Steroid saving and effective
Lever & Schaumburg-Lever[49]	1984	21	100 mg/d	Safe and effective, disease control in 21
Aberer et al[16]	1987	27	1–3 mg/kg/d	45% free of disease; 38% clinically free of disease, but with raised antibody titers; 17% with controlled disease
Tan-Lim & Bystryn[50]	1990	12	50–150 mg/d	AZA in combination with plasmapheresis decreased antibodies faster than without plasmapheresis
Mourellou et al[51]	1995	15	100 mg/d	Remission in 14 patients, less mortality compared with steroid monotreatment
Carson et al[52]	1996	72	50–250 mg/d	AZA significantly reduced mortality, steroid sparing, 37% remission, 33% stable disease
Scully et al[53]	1999	17	1–3 mg/kg/d	Not pointed out clearly. 2 deaths reported under treatment with AZA
Ljubojevic et al[54]	2002	129	100–150 mg/d	Reduction of mortality compared with patients with steroid monotherapy
Beissert et al[18]	2006	18	2 mg/kg/d	Steroid-sparing effect of AZA similar to that of MMF. Quicker response to therapy with AZA than with MMF. No significant differences in overall outcome
Rose et al[20]	2005	11	2–2.5 mg/kg/d	Tendency in favor of AZA concerning complete remissions compared with cyclophosphamide pulse therapy
Chams-Davatchi et al[19]	2007	30	2.5 mg/kg/d	AZA most effective compared with CYP and MMF or cortisone monotherapy, but no significant differences in complete remission
Chaidemenos et al[55]	2011	19	100 mg/d	Notable steroid-sparing effect of AZA; high dose of prednisone leads significantly faster to remission than low dose of prednisone combined with AZA

Abbreviations: AZA, azathioprine; CYP, cyclophosphamide; MMF, mycophenolate mofetil; N, number of patients treated with azathioprine.

Table 3
Use of azathioprine in cicatricial pemphigoid

Investigators	Year	N	AZA Dose	Main Outcome
Dantzig[56]	1973	1	150 mg/d	Remission of disease
Braun-Falco et al[57]	1981	1	100 mg/d	Among several trials of treatment, only AZA effective
Mondino & Brown[58]	1983	9	1.5 mg/kg/d	10 of 18 eyes showed no progress
Pawlofsky et al[59]	1985	1	150 mg/d	Successful treatment
Tauber et al[60]	1991	11	2 mg/kg/d	AZA failed to control disease in 9% of cases, diaminodiphenylsulfone recommended for treatment
Lugovic et al[61]	2007	1	2 mg/kg/d	AZA effective for treatment of inflammation and blistering, but no effect on scaring

Abbreviations: AZA, azathioprine; N, number of patients treated with azathioprine.

does not possess the enzymes to convert azathioprine into its active metabolites, suggesting that the fetus might have a certain protection against azathioprine-induced cellular toxicity.[31] Most large studies have shown that azathioprine during pregnancy is tolerated, although the rate of congenital malformations seems to be 3% to 9% in infants exposed antenatally.[32] Reported malformations include myelomeningocele, preaxial polydactyly, microcephaly, thymic atrophy, hypospadias, and adrenal hypoplasia.[31,32]

SIDE EFFECTS OF AZATHIOPRINE

Azathioprine is generally well tolerated. In a study of Japanese patients (n = 114) treated with azathioprine 50 mg/d for inflammatory bowel disease, 33% developed side effects over a period of 48 months of investigation.[33] The most common side effect of azathioprine is leukopenia (white blood cells $\leq$3000/μl), with 18 (15.8%) affected patients. Of these patients, 15 experienced mild leukopenia with no necessary change of dosage. Two patients (1.8%) had severe leukopenia (<1000/μl), followed by a decrease in the dose of azathioprine. Although the mild forms of

Table 4
Use of azathioprine in juvenile pemphigus

Investigators	Year	Patients' Age (y)	N	AZA Dose	Main Outcome
Harrington et al[62]	1978	15	1	50–100 mg/d	Good response
Lynde et al[63]	1984	15	1	50–125 mg/d	Complete remission after 2.5 y
Fine et al[64]	1988	13	1	50–125 mg/d	Complete remission in combination with plasmapheresis after 12 mo
Wananukul & Pongprasit[65]	1999	11–14	3	2 mg/kg/d	2 patients, controlled disease; 1 patient, complete remission
Harangi et al[66]	2001	10	1	2 mg/kg/d	After 4.5 y of treatment, complete remission

Abbreviations: AZA, azathioprine; N, number of patients treated with azathioprine.

leukopenia occurred after an average treatment period of 13.7 months (mean; range 1–47 months), the severe forms of leukopenia occurred in less than 1 month.

The next common side effects were gastrointestinal disturbances, including vomiting, nausea, and diarrhea. Eleven patients (9.6%) experienced such symptoms, which occurred shortly (<1 month) after initiation of therapy and were all self-limited after a few days. Further side effects were elevated liver function test results. One patient (0.9%) had a severe increase in liver enzyme levels with more than 20-fold increase of transaminases levels compared to normal levels after 2 weeks of treatment. After azathioprine had been discontinued, liver enzymes returned to normal levels. Three patients (2.6%) had flulike symptoms (ie, fever, headache, rash, arthralgia, myalgia, and malaise) that were self-limited after discontinuation of azathioprine. Two more patients showed mild loss of hair that did not lead to discontinuation of therapy.

The side effects observed in the Japanese patients were identical to those observed in white patients but developed after half the azathioprine dose that leads to similar side effects in white patients. Japanese patients showed TPMT gene polymorphisms less frequently compared with white patients or Africans. Although, for instance, TPMT activity–reducing TPMT*3A alleles were detected in 4.5% of British white patients, Kumagai and colleagues[34] could not find any individual in a cohort of 522 Japanese patients who carried that allele. **Table 5** shows the frequency of variant TPMT alleles in different ethnic populations. The most frequent TPMT gene polymorphisms can be found in Africans and white patients, whereas Asians have a low prevalence of TPMT gene polymorphisms. In white patients, approximately 1 in 300 patients has a distinctly reduced TPMT activity, and about 11% of white patients show a moderately reduced activity, resulting in increased production of toxic metabolites (eg, thioinosine monophosphates) when taking azathioprine.[35] Myelosuppression in patients with reduced TPMT activity develops more rapidly.[36] Uchiyama and colleagues[8] examined the relationship between the incidence of azathioprine-associated adverse effects and either the incidence of TPMT or ITPA gene polymorphisms (for the metabolic mechanism of ITPA see **Fig. 2**). In 5 of 6 patients who had developed an acute bone marrow toxicity, a mutation (94C>A) of the ITPA gene was detectable. About 75% of patients with agranulocytosis had the 94C>A allele. In red blood cells of patients with the homozygous 94C>A missense mutation, ITPA activity was below detectable levels. The frequency of 94C>A alleles was 31 of 200 in Japanese individuals (15.5%), which is

Table 5
Frequency of variant TPMT alleles in different ethnic populations

Population	n	TPMT*2 (%)	TPMT*3A (%)	TPMT*3C (%)
British	398	0.5	4.5	0.3
French	382	0.5	5.7	0.8
Americans	282	0.2	3.2	0.2
South-west Asians	198	0	1	0
African Americans	248	0.4	0.8	2.4
Kenyans	202	0	0	5.4
Ghanaians	434	0	0	7.6
Chinese	384	0	0	2.3
Japanese	1044	0	0	1.6

Abbreviation: n, number of alleles.
Adapted from Kumagai K, Hiyama K, Ishioka S, et al. Allelotype frequency of the thiopurine methyltransferase (TPMT) gene in Japanese. Pharmacogenetics 2001;11(3):277.

2.6-fold higher than in white patients.[8,37] Because of the high correlation between the side effects of azathioprine therapy and the prevalence of ITPA polymorphism genes in Japanese, it is suggested that in Japanese patients, instead of determination of TPMT gene polymorphisms or activity, a screen for ITPA gene mutations or activity should be introduced.[8] In white patients and Africans, monitoring for deficiency in TPMT activity is recommended before azathioprine is introduced.

With regard to the observed side effects of azathioprine, laboratory monitoring, including blood cell counts and serum analysis (especially liver enzymes), is recommended weekly for the first 8 weeks of treatment. After 8 weeks of treatment, the interval of laboratory monitoring can be extended to once per month.

The acute toxicity of azathioprine is low. A renal transplant patient who received a massive single overdose of azathioprine of 7500 mg experienced nausea, vomiting, and diarrhea followed by mild leukopenia, mild abnormalities in liver functions, as well as improved renal function.[38]

Like all immunosuppressive drugs, long-term intake of azathioprine raises the risk of immunosuppression-induced malignancies. In a large 20-year follow-up study, patients with rheumatoid arthritis receiving azathioprine had a 10-fold increased risk for developing immunosuppression-associated myeloproliferative disorders compared with the general population. Patients with rheumatoid arthritis without a history of azathioprine treatment had only a 5-fold increased risk of developing myeloproliferative disorders.[39] The risk of developing nonmelanoma skin cancers ([NMSCs]; SCCs and basal cell carcinomas [BCCs]) was 2-fold increased in the azathioprine-treated group with rheumatoid arthritis compared with the general population. There was a significant increase in cancer development in relation to the cumulative lifetime intake of azathioprine. In 8.6% of the patients with a lifetime intake of up to 50 g azathioprine, different kinds of cancer developed within 20 years. In patients with a cumulative dose of 200 g azathioprine, different kinds of cancer developed in more than 20% of cases within 20 years.[39]

There is strong evidence for an additive carcinogenic effect of UV radiation, especially UV-A (320–400 nm), in combination with azathioprine treatment concerning the development of NMSCs. Ramsay and colleagues[40] examined transplant recipients of Fitzpatrick skin types I to IV. From 361 patients, 187 (51.8%) developed histologically diagnosed NMSCs. The ratio of SCC to BCC was reversed in these patients from 1:3.7 before transplantation to 2:1 after transplantation.[40] NMSC increased with the duration of medical immunosuppression. Among the transplant recipients, 29.1% developed 1 or more NMSCs when immunosuppression did not exceed 5 years, but immunosuppression for 10 to 20 years led to an incidence of 72.4% of NMSCs in the treated patients. However, the patients received not only azathioprine (on average 100 mg daily) but also 225 mg of cyclosporine and 7 mg of prednisone daily (follow-up 7.1 years).

Most of the observed NMSCs in immunosuppressed transplant recipients developed on sun-exposed areas (80% of SCCs, 71% of BCCs, and 64% of keratoacanthomata). One of the active metabolites of azathioprine is thioguanine nucleotides. These nucleotides are precursors for 6-thioguanine, which can be incorporated into DNA on replication. Normally, DNA does not significantly absorb UV-A wavelengths (320–400 nm), whereas thiopurines do. 6-Thioguanine nucleotides have an absorbance maximum at 342 nm.[41] Moreover, 6-mercaptopurine as a metabolite of azathioprine generates reactive oxygen species (ROS) when exposed to UV-A.[42] O'Donovan and colleagues[41] demonstrated that biologically relevant doses of UV-A generate ROS in cultured cells with 6-thioguanine–substituted DNA. In experimental cell lines (HCT116, human colorectal carcinoma cells) containing about 0.01% 6-thioguanine–substituted DNA, irradiation with a nontoxic dose of 1 kJ/m^2 UV-A led to a 3-fold increase in adenine phos-phoribosyltransferase (*aprt*) mutation frequencies compared with nonsubstituted DNA. Neither 6-thioguanine nor UV-A alone was detectably mutagenic. In normal DNA without substitutes, 500 kJ/m^2 of UV-A irradiation was required to induce a similar increase in *aprt* mutation frequency. O'Donovan and colleagues[41] measured the amount of 6-thiogua-nine in DNA extracted from clinically normal skin of 3 azathioprine-treated patients. Around 0.02% of 6-thioguanine–substituted DNA was found. In a control group of patients who did not receive azathioprine, no substituted DNA was detectable. Further-more, azathioprine-treated patients showed a reduction of the minimal erythema dose for UV-A but not for UV-B. These findings indicate that the mutagenic effect of UV radi-ation is increased under azathioprine treatment. UV-A seems to play a more important role for photocarcinogenesis in these patients than UV-B.

In a mouse model, Reeve and colleagues[43] showed that azathioprine but not cyclo-phosphamide increased the incidence of skin tumors significantly after UV irradiation. Based on these results, it is recommended that patients undergoing therapy with azathioprine should use effective sunscreens and avoid unnecessary long-term expo-sure to the sun. Patients who require long-term treatment with azathioprine should undergo a clinical examination of the skin twice a year.

SUMMARY

Although there are still no standard guidelines for the treatment of autoimmune blis-tering diseases, azathioprine has shown good efficacy in acquired autoimmune blis-tering diseases. Azathioprine is normally well tolerated. Side effects of azathioprine normally occur in mild variants. Severe reactions are often caused by reduced TPMT or ITPA activity. Therefore, screening for the activity of TPMT should be conducted in white patients and Africans, whereas the Japanese should be screened for the activity of ITPA before therapy with azathioprine is started. Due to its potential steroid-sparing effect and the relatively rare side effects, azathioprine is clinically meaningful for the treatment of pemphigus, and recent developments in tar-geting B cells in autoimmune blistering disorders must prove their superiority against azathioprine.

REFERENCES

1. Elion GB. The purine path to chemotherapy. Science 1989;244(4900):41–7.
2. Burchenal JH, Murphy ML, Ellison RR, et al. Clinical evaluation of a new antime-tabolite, 6-mercaptopurine, in the treatment of leukemia and allied diseases. Blood 1953;8(11):965–99.
3. Calne RY. The rejection of renal homografts. Inhibition in dogs by 6-mercaptopu-rine. Lancet 1960;1(7121):417–8.
4. Calne RY, Murray JE. Inhibition of the rejection of renal homografts in dogs by Burroughs Wellcome 57–322. Surg Forum 1961;12:118–20.
5. Calne RY, Loughridge LW, Pryse-Davies J, et al. Renal transplantation in man: a report of five cases, using cadaveric donors. BMJ 1963;2(5358):645–51.
6. Berlit P. Azathioprin, internist. Praxis 1995;35:661–5.
7. Karran P, Attard N. Thiopurines in current medical practice: molecular mecha-nisms and contributions to therapy-related cancer. Nat Rev Cancer 2008;8(1): 24–36.
8. Uchiyama K, Nakamura M, Kubota T, et al. Thiopurine S-methyltransferase and inosine triphosphate pyrophosphohydrolase genes in Japanese patients with

inflammatory bowel disease in whom adverse drug reactions were induced by azathioprine/6-mercaptopurine treatment. J Gastroenterol 2009;44(3):197–203.

9. Szawlowski PW, Al-Safi SA, Dooley T, et al. Azathioprine suppresses the mixed lymphocyte reaction of patients with Lesch-Nyhan syndrome. Br J Clin Pharmacol 1985;20(5):489–91.

10. Greaves MW, Burton JL, Marks J, et al. Azathioprine in treatment of bullous pemphigoid. BMJ 1971;1(5741):144–5.

11. Burton JL, Harman RR, Peachey RD, et al. Azathioprine plus prednisone in treatment of pemphigoid. BMJ 1978;2(6146):1190–1.

12. Guillaume JC, Vaillant L, Bernard P, et al. Controlled trial of azathioprine and plasma exchange in addition to prednisolone in the treatment of bullous pemphigoid. Arch Dermatol 1993;129(1):49–53.

13. Beissert S, Werfel T, Frieling U, et al. A comparison of oral methylprednisolone plus azathioprine or mycophenolate mofetil for the treatment of bullous pemphigoid. Arch Dermatol 2007;143(12):1536–42.

14. Kirtschig G, Middleton P, Bennett C, et al. Interventions for bullous pemphigoid [review]. Cochrane Database Syst Rev 2010;10:CD002292.

15. Krakowski A, Covo J, Rozanski Z. Pemphigus vulgaris. Arch Dermatol 1969; 100(1):117.

16. Aberer W, Wolff-Schreiner EC, Stingl G, et al. Azathioprine in the treatment of pemphigus vulgaris. A long-term follow-up. J Am Acad Dermatol 1987;16(3 Pt 1): 527–33.

17. Lever WF, Schaumburg-Lever G. Immunosuppressants and prednisone in pemphigus vulgaris: therapeutic results obtained in 63 patients between 1961 and 1975. Arch Dermatol 1977;113(9):1236–41.

18. Beissert S, Werfel T, Frieling U, et al. A comparison of oral methylprednisolone plus azathioprine or mycophenolate mofetil for the treatment of pemphigus. Arch Dermatol 2006;142(11):1447–54.

19. Chams-Davatchi C, Esmaili N, Daneshpazhooh M, et al. Randomized controlled open-label trial of four treatment regimens for pemphigus vulgaris. J Am Acad Dermatol 2007;57(4):622–8.

20. Rose E, Wever S, Zilliken D, et al. Intravenous dexamethasone-cyclophosphamide pulse therapy in comparison with oral methylprednisolone-azathioprine therapy in patients with pemphigus: results of a multicenter prospectively randomized study. J Dtsch Dermatol Ges 2005;3(3):200–6.

21. Zillikens D, Miller K, Hartmann AA, et al. IgA pemphigus foliaceus: a case report. Dermatologica 1990;181(4):304–7.

22. Monshi B, Marker M, Feichtinger H, et al. Pemphigus vegetans–immunopathological findings in a rare variant of pemphigus v vulgaris. J Dtsch Dermatol Ges 2010;8(3):179–83.

23. Faulde MK, Sorhage B, Ksoll A, et al. Complete remission of drug resistant Pemphigus vegetans treated by extracorporeal photopheresis. J Eur Acad Dermatol Venereol 2007;21:822–49.

24. Ichimiya M, Yamamoto K, Muto M. Successful treatment of pemphigus vegetans by addition of etretinate to systemic steroids. Clin Exp Dermatol 1998;23(4): 178–80.

25. Kimyai-Asadi A, Jih MH. Paraneoplastic pemphigus. Int J Dermatol 2001;40(6): 367–72.

26. Lam S, Stone MS, Goeken JA, et al. Paraneoplastic pemphigus, cicatricial conjunctivitis, and acanthosis nigricans with pachydermatoglyphy in a patient with bronchogenic squamous cell carcinoma. Ophthalmology 1992;99(1):108–13.

27. Verrini A, Cannata G, Cozzani E, et al. A patient with immunological features of paraneoplastic pemphigus in the absence of a detectable malignancy. Acta Derm Venereol 2002;82(5):382–4.
28. Martin LK, Agero AL, Werth V, et al. Interventions for pemphigus vulgaris and pemphigus foliaceus. Cochrane Database Syst Rev 2009;1:CD006263. DOI: 10.1002/14651858.CD006263.pub2.
29. Mensing H, Brehm H, Nasemann T. Bullöses Pemphigoid im Kindesalter. Hautarzt 1984;35:254–8 [in German].
30. Ostensen M. Treatment with immunosuppressive and disease modifying drugs during pregnancy and lactation [review]. Am J Reprod Immunol 1992;28(3–4): 148–52.
31. Janssen NM, Genta MS. The effects of immunosuppressive and anti-inflammatory medications on fertility, pregnancy, and lactation. Arch Intern Med 2000;160(5): 610–9.
32. Tendron A, Gouyon JB, Decramer S. In utero exposure to immunosuppressive drugs: experimental and clinical studies. Pediatr Nephrol 2002;17(2):121–30.
33. Takatsu N, Matsui T, Murakami Y, et al. Adverse reactions to azathioprine cannot be predicted by thiopurine S-methyltransferase genotype in Japanese patients with inflammatory bowel disease. J Gastroenterol Hepatol 2009;24(7):1258–64.
34. Kumagai K, Hiyama K, Ishioka S, et al. Allelotype frequency of the thiopurine methyltransferase (TPMT) gene in Japanese. Pharmacogenetics 2001;11(3):275–8.
35. Lennard L, Van Loon JA, Weinshilboum RM. Pharmacogenetics of acute azathioprine toxicity: relationship to thiopurine methyltransferase genetic polymorphism. Clin Pharmacol Ther 1989;46(2):149–54.
36. Anstey A, Lennard L, Mayou SC, et al. Pancytopenia related to azathioprine–an enzyme deficiency caused by a common genetic polymorphism: a review. J R Soc Med 1992;85(12):752–6.
37. Sumi S, Marinaki AM, Arenas M, et al. Genetic basis of inosine triphosphate pyrophosphohydrolase deficiency. Hum Genet 2002;111(4–5):360–7.
38. Carney DM, Zukoski CF, Ogden DA. Massive azathioprine overdose. Case report and review of the literature. Am J Med 1974;56(1):133–6.
39. Silman AJ, Petrie J, Hazleman B, et al. Lymphoproliferative cancer and other malignancy in patients with rheumatoid arthritis treated with azathioprine: a 20 year follow up study. Ann Rheum Dis 1988;47(12):988–92.
40. Ramsay HM, Fryer AA, Hawley CM, et al. Non-melanoma skin cancer risk in the Queensland renal transplant population. Br J Dermatol 2002;147(5):950–6.
41. O'Donovan P, Perrett CM, Zhang X, et al. Azathioprine and UVA light generate mutagenic oxidative DNA damage. Science 2005;309:1871–4.
42. Hemmens VJ, Moore DE. Photochemical sensitization by azathioprine and its metabolites–I. 6-Mercaptopurine. Photochem Photobiol 1986;43(3):247–55.
43. Reeve VE, Greenoak GE, Gallagher CH, et al. Effect of immunosuppressive agents and sunscreens on UV carcinogenesis in the hairless mouse. Aust J Exp Biol Med Sci 1985;63(Pt 6):655–65.
44. van Dijk TJ, van Velde JL. Treatment of pemphigus and pemphigoid with azathioprine. Dermatologica 1973;147(3):179–85.
45. Burton JL, Greaves MW. Azathioprine for pemphigus and pemphigoid–a 4 year follow-up. Br J Dermatol 1974;91(1):103–9.
46. Ahmed AR, Maize JC, Provost TT. Bullous pemphigoid. Clinical and immunologic follow-up after successful therapy. Arch Dermatol 1977;113(8):1043–6.
47. Burton JL, Greaves MW, Marks J, et al. Azathioprine in pemphigus vulgaris. BMJ 1970;3(5714):84–6.

48. Roenigk HH Jr, Deodhar S. Pemphigus treatment with azathioprine. Clinical and immunologic correlation. Arch Dermatol 1973;107(3):353–7.
49. Lever WF, Schaumburg-Lever G. Treatment of pemphigus vulgaris. Results obtained in 84 patients between 1961 and 1982. Arch Dermatol 1984;120(1):44–7.
50. Tan-Lim R, Bystryn JC. Effect of plasmapheresis therapy on circulating levels of pemphigus antibodies. J Am Acad Dermatol 1990;22(1):35–40.
51. Mourellou O, Chaidemenos GC, Koussidou T, et al. The treatment of pemphigus vulgaris. Experience with 48 patients seen over an 11-year period. Br J Dermatol 1995;133(1):83–7.
52. Carson PJ, Hameed A, Ahmed AR. Influence of treatment on the clinical course of pemphigus vulgaris. J Am Acad Dermatol 1996;34(4):645–52.
53. Scully C, Paes De Almeida O, Porter SR, et al. Pemphigus vulgaris: the manifestations and long-term management of 55 patients with oral lesions. Br J Dermatol 1999;140(1):84–9.
54. Ljubojević S, Lipozencić J, Brenner S, et al. Pemphigus vulgaris: a review of treatment over a 19-year period. J Eur Acad Dermatol Venereol 2002;16(6):599–603.
55. Chaidemenos G, Apalla Z, Koussidou T, et al. High dose oral prednisone vs. prednisone plus azathioprine for the treatment of oral pemphigus: a retrospective, bi-centre, comparative study. J Eur Acad Dermatol Venereol 2011;25(2):206–10.
56. Dantzig P. Circulating antibodies in cicatricial pemphigoid. Arch Dermatol 1973; 108(2):264–6.
57. Braun-Falco O, Wolff HH, Ponce E. Disseminated cicatricial pemphigoid. Hautarzt 1981;32(5):233–9.
58. Mondino BJ, Brown SI. Immunosuppressive therapy in ocular cicatricial pemphigoid. Am J Ophthalmol 1983;96(4):453–9.
59. Pawlofsky C, Simon M Jr, Fartasch M, et al. Disseminated cicatricial pemphigoid. Dermatologica 1985;171(4):259–63.
60. Tauber J, Sainz de la Maza M, Foster CS. Systemic chemotherapy for ocular cicatricial pemphigoid. Cornea 1991;10(3):185–95.
61. Lugović L, Buljan M, Situm M, et al. Unrecognized cicatricial pemphigoid with oral manifestations and ocular complications. A case report. Acta Dermatovenerol Croat 2007;15(4):236–42.
62. Harrington I, Sneddon IB, Walker AE. Pemphigus vulgaris in a 15-year-old girl. Acta Derm Venereol 1978;58(3):277–9.
63. Lynde CW, Ongley RC, Rigg JM. Juvenile pemphigus vulgaris. Arch Dermatol 1984;120(8):1098–9.
64. Fine JD, Appell ML, Green LK, et al. Pemphigus vulgaris. Combined treatment with intravenous corticosteroid pulse therapy, plasmapheresis, and azathioprine. Arch Dermatol 1988;124(2):236–9.
65. Wananukul S, Pongprasit P. Childhood pemphigus. Int J Dermatol 1999;38(1): 29–35.
66. Harangi F, Várszegi D, Schneider I, et al. Complete recovery from juvenile pemphigus vulgaris. Pediatr Dermatol 2001;18(1):51–3.

Mycophenolate Mofetil for the Management of Autoimmune Bullous Diseases

Marina Eskin-Schwartz, MD, PhD[a,b], Michael David, MD[a,b],
Daniel Mimouni, MD[a,b],*

KEYWORDS

- Mycophenolate mofetil • Autoimmune bullous diseases
- Immunosuppression • Mycophenolic acid

Mycophenolate mofetil (MMF) is the 2-morpholinoethyl ester of mycophenolic acid (MPA), one of the several phenol compounds first described by Alsberg and Black in 1913 in cultures of *Penicillium stoloniferum*. MPA has been found to inhibit DNA synthesis by selectively inhibiting inosine monophosphate dehydrogenase (IMPDH), an enzyme that catalyzes the rate-limiting step in the de novo biosynthesis of guanine nucleotides (reviewed in Ref.[1]). MPA targets mainly T and B lymphocytes which, unlike other cell types, are dependent almost exclusively on the de novo guanine nucleotide synthesis pathway for proliferation and differentiation.[2] MPA is a fivefold more potent inhibitor of the IMPDH II isoform specific to lymphocytes than of the housekeeping IMPDH I isoform, found in most cell types.[3] MMF inhibits T and B cell proliferation,[4] induces apoptosis of T cells,[5] and inhibits antibody production by B cells.[6]

Besides its antiproliferative effect on lymphocytes, MMF has several other mechanisms of action. Guanosine triphosphate (GTP) depletion caused by MMF impairs fucosylation and surface expression of adhesion molecules of lymphocytes and monocytes, preventing their attachment to endothelial cells during their recruitment to inflammation sites.[7,8] As monocytes and macrophages are major producers of proinflammatory cytokines causing fibroblast recruitment and proliferation at the

---

A version of this article was previously published in *Dermatologic Clinics 29:4*.

Disclosure: The authors have no financial interest in this article.

[a] Department of Dermatology, Rabin Medical Center, Beilinson Campus, Jabotinski Street 39, Petah Tiqwa 49100, Israel; [b] Department of Dermatology, Sackler Faculty of Medicine, Tel Aviv University, PO Box 39040, Tel Aviv 69978, Israel

* Corresponding author. Department of Dermatology, Rabin Medical Center, Beilinson Campus, Jabotinski Street 39, Petah Tiqwa 49100, Israel.

E-mail address: mimouni@post.tau.ac.il

inflammation site (such as tumor necrosis factor α and interleukin-1), their depletion reduces production of these cytokines, inhibiting fibroblast proliferation and tissue fibrosis.[9] MPA was shown to inhibit the surface expression of antigens responsible for maturation and efficient antigen presentation by dendritic cells, thereby suppressing immune responses.[10,11] GTP depletion also impairs inducible nitric oxide synthase (iNOS) activity, which leads to a reduction of the oxidative stress caused by activated monocytes, macrophages, and endothelial cells.[12]

MMF has 94% oral bioavailability.[13] Following absorption MMF is converted to its active metabolite, MPA, by plasma, liver, and kidney esterases. MPA is almost completely inactivated in the liver by glucuronyl transferase,[14] and a significant portion of MPA-glucuronide (MPAG) is secreted into the bile and recycled via enterohepatic recirculation. MPAG is converted back to MPA by β-glucuronidase, found mainly in the epidermis and the gastrointestinal tract. The peak plasma level of the drug is reached in less than 1 hour; the elimination rate is 18 hours. A secondary MPA peak occurs at 6 to 12 hours, due to the enterohepatic circulation.[15] Ninety-seven percent of MPA is albumin bound. Most of the drug is excreted as MPAG in the urine.[13]

The most common side effects of MMF are nausea, vomiting, abdominal cramps, and diarrhea, reported in 12% to 36% of patients.[16] All are dose dependent. Hematologic side effects, also dose dependent and reversible upon discontinuation of the drug, include leukopenia, neutropenia, and thrombocytopenia. There are reports of genitourinary side effects of urgency, frequency, dysuria, and sterile pyuria, which generally resolve with continued drug use.[17] Neurologic complaints (headache, tinnitus, and insomnia), rash, and cardiovascular effects (peripheral edema and hypertension) have also been described. MPA/MMF treatment has been associated with an increased incidence of both bacterial and viral infections (especially herpes zoster[17,18] and cytomegalovirus[19–21]). Of importance, a risk of cytomegalovirus infection has been reported in organ transplant patients given MPA/MMF, concomitantly treated with other immunosuppressive agents. The ability of MMF to induce malignancy is controversial. MMF is expected to be less carcinogenic than azathioprine because it is not incorporated into the DNA and does not cause chromosomal breaks.[22] Some studies reported a dose-dependent increase in the risk of lymphoproliferative malignancy in MMF-treated organ transplant patients,[23–25] but this finding was not supported in a comparative study of MMF-based and other immunosuppressive regimens in renal transplant patients.[26] In dermatologic literature an early report described 3 cases of malignancy during MMF treatment in psoriatic patients.[27] Subsequently, Epinette and colleagues[17] found no increase in the incidence of cancer in psoriatic patients treated with MMF.

A limited number of cases reports suggested MMF could cause fetal malformations in humans.[27,28] MMF is classified as pregnancy category D (ie, there is positive evidence of human fetal risk based on adverse reaction data from investigational or marketing experience or studies in humans, but potential benefits may warrant use of the drug in pregnant women despite potential risks), and therefore it is recommended to use two different reliable methods of birth control 4 weeks before starting and during MMF therapy, and continue birth control for 6 weeks after stopping MMF.

Several drugs are known to interact with MMF via mechanisms of absorption inhibition (antacids), disruption of enterohepatic recirculation (antibiotics, cholestyramine), albumin binding (phenytoin, salicylic acid), and prevention of kidney tubular secretion of MPA (acyclovir, gancyclovir, probenecid).[29,30]

MPA was first used in dermatology in the 1970s as an anti-inflammatory agent to treat moderate to severe psoriasis.[31,32] However, by the end of the decade its use was discontinued owing to its gastrointestinal side effects, increased risk of latent viral infections, and possible carcinogenicity.[27] A decade later MMF, the 2-morpholinoethyl ester of MPA, received approval from the from the Food and Drug Administration as an immunosuppressive agent in renal transplant patients, with studies showing that it had better oral bioavailability than MPA and caused fewer gastrointestinal side effects. Owing to its long-term safety and tolerability, it began to be applied in other fields, including dermatology.

Autoimmune bullous diseases are a group of blistering disorders that share a pathogenetic mechanism of autoantibody production against different epidermal and dermoepidermal junction proteins. High-dose steroids are the traditional first-line treatment, but their multiple and potentially severe side effects with prolonged use have prompted dermatologists to seek alternative or steroid-sparing agents. Today, immunosuppressive agents such as azathioprine, cyclophosphamide, and MMF are widely used in the treatment of these diseases.

The initial evidence of the benefit of MMF for pemphigus stems from several case series, reporting the efficacy of MMF as a steroid-sparing agent.

Enk and Knop[33] combined MMF (2 g/d) with prednisolone (2 mg/kg/d) in 12 patients with pemphigus vulgaris, who had relapsed during azathioprine and prednisolone therapy. Eleven patients responded to this therapy, with no relapses during the 9- to 12-month follow-up period. A similar regimen was applied by Chams-Davatchi and colleagues[34] in 10 patients with pemphigus vulgaris with severe resistant/recurrent disease. The lesions completely cleared in 9 patients by 6 to 16 weeks. Five patients relapsed after MMF discontinuation at 6 months' follow-up, suggesting MMF should be administered for a longer period to sustain remission. Several years later, a large historical prospective trial was conducted that included 31 patients with pemphigus vulgaris and 11 patients with pemphigus foliaceus, who had relapsed on prednisone therapy or had had adverse effects from previous drug therapy.[35] Treatment with MMF (35–45 mg/kg) combined with prednisone led to complete remission in 71% of the pemphigus vulgaris group and 45% of the pemphigus foliaceus group. Mean time to remission was 9 months, and the remission was maintained throughout the 22 months of follow-up.

Powell and colleagues[36] reported treating 16 refractory pemphigus vulgaris and pemphigus foliaceus patients with MMF (starting at 500 mg/d and increasing as tolerated) and prednisone. Clinically inactive disease was achieved in 7 patients. The much lower doses of prednisone at the time of MMF initiation in this study are noteworthy, and may explain the relatively low rate of clinical remission.

In a prospective study of MMF as first-line treatment, Esmaili and colleagues[37] administered MMF (2 g/d) and prednisolone (2 mg/kg/d) to 31 patients with pemphigus vulgaris, with a 12-month follow-up. MMF was beneficial in 21 patients (67.7%), and its addition made it possible to taper down the prednisolone, suggesting its value as a steroid-sparing agent. A more recent prospective controlled trial was conducted by Beissert and colleagues,[38] who randomized 96 patients with mild to moderate pemphigus vulgaris to receive MMF (2–3 g/d) plus prednisolone or placebo plus prednisolone. At the end of the 52-week follow-up, a similar treatment response rate was observed in the two groups. The patients given MMF showed faster and more durable responses, but this difference may have been attributable to the milder disease of the placebo group, which may not have needed the additional immunosuppressive therapy. In all the aforementioned studies the MMF therapy was well tolerated. The most common side effects were gastrointestinal complaints, lymphopenia, and bacterial and viral infections.[33–38]

MMF/mycophenolate sodium monotherapy for pemphigus vulgaris has shown variable success in several case series.[39,40]

Several randomized open-label trials compared the efficacy of MMF as a steroid-sparing agent with other immunosuppressive drugs in patients with pemphigus. Beissert and colleagues[41] treated 40 patients with pemphigus vulgaris or pemphigus foliaceus with methylprednisolone and azathioprine or methylprednisolone and MMF. There was no difference between MMF and azathioprine in efficacy, steroid-sparing effect, or safety profile.

In a random controlled study Chams-Davatchi and colleagues[42] compared 4 treatment regimens in 120 patients with pemphigus vulgaris: prednisolone only, prednisolone and azathioprine, prednisolone and MMF, and prednisolone and intravenous cyclophosphamide pulse therapy. There was no difference in complete remission rate between the groups (70%–80% of patients). All immunosuppressive drugs had a steroid-sparing effect; the most efficacious was azathioprine, followed by pulse cyclophosphamide and then MMF.

A few patients with paraneoplastic pemphigus were reported to benefit from combined immunosuppressive regimens, including MMF and corticosteroids[36] or MMF, corticosteroids, and azathioprine.[43]

Several case reports suggested that MMF, alone or combined with corticosteroids, is effective for the treatment of bullous pemphigoid.[39,44,45]

A large, prospective, randomized trial of 73 patients with bullous pemphigoid found MMF to be equally efficacious to azathioprine in inducing disease remission (100%) when combined with corticosteroids.[46] Although the average time to complete remission was shorter in the azathioprine-treated group, the MMF group had less liver toxicity.

Enteric-coated mycophenolate sodium (EC-MPS)/MMF has also been used as a steroid-sparing agent[47,48] or in combination with dapsone[49] for the treatment of cicatricial pemphigoid. Two retrospective studies addressed the role of MMF in the treatment of ocular cicatricial pemphigoid. Daniel and colleagues[50] reported successful control of eye inflammation at 1 year in 70% of 18 patients treated with MMF and prednisone. Saw and colleagues[51] retrospectively compared various immunosuppressive drugs in 115 patients with ocular cicatricial pemphigoid, and found cyclophosphamide to be more successful (69%) than mycophenolate (59%) in controlling the inflammation. However, mycophenolate had the fewest side effects of all the drugs used in the study.

MMF has shown variable success in individual patients with epidermolysis bullosa acquisita.[52–54] Similarly, several case reports suggested that MMF and EC-MPS were effective for the treatment of refractory linear IgA disease[55–57] and linear IgA bullous dermatosis of childhood.[58]

In summary, MMF is an immunosuppressive drug widely used today in multiple fields of medicine, including dermatology. Advantages of MMF include its wide therapeutic index, mild side effects, and lack of major end-organ toxicity. MMF has been successfully applied for the treatment of various autoimmune blistering diseases, including pemphigus, bullous pemphigoid, and cicatricial pemphigoid, mostly as a steroid-sparing agent. According to numerous case series, MMF could be of value in treating refractory disease. The few randomized clinical trials conducted to date of patients with pemphigus and bullous pemphigoid report a similar efficacy for MMF to other immunosuppressants. Large-scale clinical trials are needed to further delineate the value of MMF in this setting.

REFERENCES

1. Allison AC. Mechanisms of action of mycophenolate mofetil. Lupus 2005; 14(Suppl 1):s2–8.

2. Allison AC, Eugui EM. Immunosuppressive and other effects of mycophenolic acid and an ester prodrug, mycophenolate mofetil. Immunol Rev 1993;136:5–28.

3. Carr SF, Papp E, Wu JC, et al. Characterization of human type I and type II IMP dehydrogenases. J Biol Chem 1993;268:27286–90.

4. Allison AC, Eugui EM. Mycophenolate mofetil and its mechanisms of action. Immunopharmacology 2000;47:85–118.

5. Cohn RG, Mirkovich A, Dunlap B, et al. Mycophenolic acid increases apoptosis, lysosomes and lipid droplets in human lymphoid and monocytic cell lines. Transplantation 1999;68:411–8.

6. Allison AC, Almquist SJ, Muller CD, et al. In vitro immunosuppressive effects of mycophenolic acid and an ester pro-drug, RS-61443. Transplant Proc 1991;23:10–4.

7. Allison AC, Kowalski WJ, Muller CJ, et al. Mycophenolic acid and brequinar, inhibitors of purine and pyrimidine synthesis, block the glycosylation of adhesion molecules. Transplant Proc 1993;25:67–70.

8. Blaheta RA, Leckel K, Wittig B, et al. Mycophenolate mofetil impairs transendothelial migration of allogeneic CD4 and CD8 T-cells. Transplant Proc 1999;31:1250–2.

9. Morath C, Schwenger V, Beimler J, et al. Antifibrotic actions of mycophenolic acid. Clin Transplant 2006;20(Suppl 17):25–9.

10. Colic M, Stojic-Vukanic Z, Pavlovic B, et al. Mycophenolate mofetil inhibits differentiation, maturation and allostimulatory function of human monocyte-derived dendritic cells. Clin Exp Immunol 2003;134:63–9.

11. Lagaraine C, Lebranchu Y. Effects of immunosuppressive drugs on dendritic cells and tolerance induction. Transplantation 2003;75:37S–42S.

12. Senda M, DeLustro B, Eugui E, et al. Mycophenolic acid, an inhibitor of IMP dehydrogenase that is also an immunosuppressive agent, suppresses the cytokine-induced nitric oxide production in mouse and rat vascular endothelial cells. Transplantation 1995;60:1143–8.

13. Bullingham RE, Nicholls AJ, Kamm BR. Clinical pharmacokinetics of mycophenolate mofetil. Clin Pharm 1998;34:429–55.

14. Sweeney MJ. Mycophenolic acid and its mechanism of action in cancer and psoriasis. Jpn J Antibiot 1977;30(Suppl):85–92.

15. Bullingham R, Monroe S, Nicholls A, et al. Pharmacokinetics and bioavailability of mycophenolate mofetil in healthy subjects after single-dose oral and intravenous administration. J Clin Pharmacol 1996;36:315–24.

16. Hoffman-La Roche Ltd. Cellcept (mycophenolate mofetil); 1997 [package insert]. Available at: http://www.gene.com/gene/products/information/cellcept/pdf/pi.pdf. Accessed June 24, 2011.

17. Epinette WW, Parker CM, Jones EL, et al. Mycophenolic acid for psoriasis. A review of pharmacology, long-term efficacy, and safety. J Am Acad Dermatol 1987;17:962–71.

18. Simmons WD, Rayhill SC, Sollinger HW. Preliminary risk-benefit assessment of mycophenolate mofetil in transplant rejection. Drug Saf 1997;17:75–92.

19. Hambach L, Stadler M, Dammann E, et al. Increased risk of complicated CMV infection with the use of mycophenolate mofetil in allogeneic stem cell transplantation. Bone Marrow Transplant 2002;29:903–6.

20. Sarmiento JM, Dockrell DH, Schwab TR, et al. Mycophenolate mofetil increases cytomegalovirus invasive organ disease in renal transplant patients. Clin Transplant 2000;14:136–8.

21. ter Meulen CG, Wetzels JF, Hilbrands LB. The influence of mycophenolate mofetil on the incidence and severity of primary cytomegalovirus infections and disease after renal transplantation. Nephrol Dial Transplant 2000;15:711–4.

22. Kitchin JE, Pomeranz MK, Pak G, et al. Rediscovering mycophenolic acid: a review of its mechanism, side effects, and potential uses. J Am Acad Dermatol 1997;37:445–9.
23. Mycophenolate mofetil in cadaveric renal transplantation. US Renal Transplant Mycophenolate Mofetil Study Group. Am J Kidney Dis 1999;34:296–303.
24. Mathew TH. A blinded, long-term, randomized multicenter study of mycophenolate mofetil in cadaveric renal transplantation: results at three years. Tricontinental Mycophenolate Mofetil Renal Transplantation Study Group. Transplantation 1998; 65:1450–4.
25. Mycophenolate mofetil in renal transplantation: 3-year results from the placebo-controlled trial. European Mycophenolate Mofetil Cooperative Study Group. Transplantation 1999;68:391–6.
26. Robson R, Cecka JM, Opelz G, et al. Prospective registry-based observational cohort study of the long-term risk of malignancies in renal transplant patients treated with mycophenolate mofetil. Am J Transplant 2005;5:2954–60.
27. Lynch WS, Roenigk HH Jr. Mycophenolic acid for psoriasis. Arch Dermatol 1977; 113:1203–8.
28. Anderka MT, Lin AE, Abuelo DN, et al. Reviewing the evidence for mycophenolate mofetil as a new teratogen: case report and review of the literature. Am J Med Genet A 2009;149A:1241–8.
29. Perlis C, Pan T, McDonald C. Cytotoxic agents. In: Wolverton S, editor. Comprehensive dermatologic drug therapy. Philadelphia: Elsevier; 2007. p. 1099.
30. Gimenez F, Foeillet E, Bourdon O, et al. Evaluation of pharmacokinetic interactions after oral administration of mycophenolate mofetil and valaciclovir or aciclovir to healthy subjects. Clin Pharm 2004;43:685–92.
31. Jones EL, Epinette WW, Hackney VC, et al. Treatment of psoriasis with oral mycophenolic acid. J Invest Dermatol 1975;65:537–42.
32. Gomez EC, Menendez L, Frost P. Efficacy of mycophenolic acid for the treatment of psoriasis. J Am Acad Dermatol 1979;1:531–7.
33. Enk AH, Knop J. Mycophenolate is effective in the treatment of pemphigus vulgaris. Arch Dermatol 1999;135:54–6.
34. Chams-Davatchi C, Nonahal Azar R, Daneshpazooh M, et al. Open trial of mycophenolate mofetil in the treatment of resistant pemphigus vulgaris. Ann Dermatol Venereol 2002;129:23–5 [in French].
35. Mimouni D, Anhalt GJ, Cummins DL, et al. Treatment of pemphigus vulgaris and pemphigus foliaceus with mycophenolate mofetil. Arch Dermatol 2003;139: 739–42.
36. Powell AM, Albert S, Al Fares S, et al. An evaluation of the usefulness of mycophenolate mofetil in pemphigus. Br J Dermatol 2003;149:138–45.
37. Esmaili N, Chams-Davatchi C, Valikhani M, et al. Treatment of pemphigus vulgaris with mycophenolate mofetil as a steroid-sparing agent. Eur J Dermatol 2008;18: 159–64.
38. Beissert S, Mimouni D, Kanwar AJ, et al. Treating pemphigus vulgaris with prednisone and mycophenolate mofetil: a multicenter, randomized, placebo-controlled trial. J Invest Dermatol 2010;130:2041–8.
39. Grundmann-Kollmann M, Korting HC, Behrens S, et al. Mycophenolate mofetil: a new therapeutic option in the treatment of blistering autoimmune diseases. J Am Acad Dermatol 1999;40:957–60.
40. Baskan EB, Yilmaz M, Tunali S, et al. Efficacy and safety of long-term mycophenolate sodium therapy in pemphigus vulgaris. J Eur Acad Dermatol Venereol 2009;23:1432–4.

41. Beissert S, Werfel T, Frieling U, et al. A comparison of oral methylprednisolone plus azathioprine or mycophenolate mofetil for the treatment of pemphigus. Arch Dermatol 2006;142:1447–54.
42. Chams-Davatchi C, Esmaili N, Daneshpazhooh M, et al. Randomized controlled open-label trial of four treatment regimens for pemphigus vulgaris. J Am Acad Dermatol 2007;57:622–8.
43. Williams JV, Marks JG Jr, Billingsley EM. Use of mycophenolate mofetil in the treatment of paraneoplastic pemphigus. Br J Dermatol 2000;142:506–8.
44. Bohm M, Beissert S, Schwarz T, et al. Bullous pemphigoid treated with mycophenolate mofetil. Lancet 1997;349:541.
45. Nousari HC, Griffin WA, Anhalt GJ. Successful therapy for bullous pemphigoid with mycophenolate mofetil. J Am Acad Dermatol 1998;39:497–8.
46. Beissert S, Werfel T, Frieling U, et al. A comparison of oral methylprednisolone plus azathioprine or mycophenolate mofetil for the treatment of bullous pemphigoid. Arch Dermatol 2007;143:1536–42.
47. Megahed M, Schmiedeberg S, Becker J, et al. Treatment of cicatricial pemphigoid with mycophenolate mofetil as a steroid-sparing agent. J Am Acad Dermatol 2001;45:256–9.
48. Marzano AV, Dassoni F, Caputo R. Treatment of refractory blistering autoimmune diseases with mycophenolic acid. J Dermatolog Treat 2006;17:370–6.
49. Ingen-Housz-Oro S, Prost-Squarcioni C, Pascal F, et al. Cicatricial pemphigoid: treatment with mycophenolate mofetil. Ann Dermatol Venereol 2005;132:13–6 [in French].
50. Daniel E, Thorne JE, Newcomb CW, et al. Mycophenolate mofetil for ocular inflammation. Am J Ophthalmol 2010;149:423–32.
51. Saw VP, Dart JK, Rauz S, et al. Immunosuppressive therapy for ocular mucous membrane pemphigoid strategies and outcomes. Ophthalmology 2008;115: 253–61.
52. Schattenkirchner S, Eming S, Hunzelmann N, et al. Treatment of epidermolysis bullosa acquisita with mycophenolate mofetil and autologous keratinocyte grafting. Br J Dermatol 1999;141:932–3.
53. Kowalzick L, Suckow S, Ziegler H, et al. Mycophenolate mofetil in epidermolysis bullosa acquisita. Dermatology 2003;207:332–4.
54. Tran MM, Anhalt GJ, Barrett T, et al. Childhood IgA-mediated epidermolysis bullosa acquisita responding to mycophenolate mofetil as a corticosteroid-sparing agent. J Am Acad Dermatol 2006;54:734–6.
55. Talhari C, Mahnke N, Ruzicka T, et al. Successful treatment of linear IgA disease with mycophenolate mofetil as a corticosteroid sparing agent. Clin Exp Dermatol 2005;30:297–8.
56. Lewis MA, Yaqoob NA, Emanuel C, et al. Successful treatment of oral linear IgA disease using mycophenolate. Oral Surg Oral Med Oral Pathol Oral Radiol Endod 2007;103:483–6.
57. Marzano AV, Ramoni S, Spinelli D, et al. Refractory linear IgA bullous dermatosis successfully treated with mycophenolate sodium. J Dermatolog Treat 2008;19: 364–7.
58. Farley-Li J, Mancini AJ. Treatment of linear IgA bullous dermatosis of childhood with mycophenolate mofetil. Arch Dermatol 2003;139:1121–4.

Dapsone in the Management of Autoimmune Bullous Diseases

Evan W. Piette, MD[a], Victoria P. Werth, MD[a,b],*

KEYWORDS

• Dapsone • Autoimmune bullous disease • Review

Dapsone is a sulfone-derived medication that was first used in humans to treat leprosy in the 1940s.[1] Since then, it has been used as an antimicrobial agent and has been found to have antiinflammatory properties. Dapsone is used in several dermatologic conditions, particularly those with neutrophil predominance because it inhibits neutrophil activation and recruitment through several different pathways.[1] Dapsone has also been used in the treatment of the autoimmune bullous diseases (AIBD), a group of disorders resulting from autoimmunity directed against basement membrane and/or intercellular adhesion molecules on cutaneous and mucosal surfaces.[2] This review summarizes the published data evaluating dapsone as a therapy for AIBD. Common adverse effects of this medication include methemoglobinemia and anemia, particularly in patients who are glucose-6-phosphate dehydrogenase deficient. There are also several additional rare adverse effects associated with dapsone use, notably agranulocytosis and a hypersensitivity reaction known as the dapsone syndrome.[1,2]

PEMPHIGUS

Pemphigus is an antibody-mediated blistering disease that primarily affects the elderly and is associated with high morbidity and, when untreated, mortality. Two subtypes of pemphigus are reviewed here: pemphigus vulgaris (PV) and pemphigus foliaceus (PF). Immunosuppressives are the mainstay of treatment of PV, and dapsone was first reported as an adjunct to therapy in the 1960s.[3] There has been 1 randomized,

A version of this article was previously published in *Dermatologic Clinics 29:4*.

Funding: National Institutes of Health, including NIH K24-AR 02207 (V.P.W.).

[a] Department of Dermatology, Perelman Center for Advanced Medicine, Suite 1-330A, 3400 Civic Center Boulevard, Philadelphia, PA 19104, USA; [b] Division of Dermatology, Philadelphia V.A. Medical Center, Philadelphia, PA, USA

* Corresponding author. Department of Dermatology, Perelman Center for Advanced Medicine, Suite 1-330A, 3400 Civic Center Boulevard, Philadelphia, PA 19104.

E-mail address: werth@mail.med.upenn.edu

Immunol Allergy Clin N Am 32 (2012) 317–322

doi:10.1016/j.iac.2012.04.011 immunology.theclinics.com

double-blind, placebo-controlled trial evaluating the use of dapsone for PV.[4,5] In this study by Werth and colleagues,[4] 19 patients receiving systemic immunosuppressive therapy for PV were randomized to 2 groups treated with the addition of either dapsone or placebo. Success was defined by the ability to taper systemic glucocorticoids to at least 7.5 mg/d within 1 year of reaching the maximum dose of dapsone (200 mg/d). Of the 9 patients receiving dapsone, 5 (56%) were successfully treated, 3 failed treatment, and 1 dropped out of the study. Of the 10 patients receiving placebo, 3 (30%) were successfully treated and 7 failed treatment. Although the difference between groups was not significant ($P = .37$), the trend favored the dapsone-treated group. In addition, 4 patients in the placebo group failed treatment and were switched to treatment with dapsone. Of these, 3 (75%) were successfully treated after initiating dapsone. Overall, 8 of 11 patients (73%) receiving dapsone versus 3 of 10 (30%) receiving placebo reached the primary outcome measure of 7.5 mg/d or less of prednisone. No adverse events requiring the discontinuation of dapsone were noted.[4]

The remaining published data on dapsone for pemphigus stem from case reports and series, nicely summarized in a 2009 review by Gürcan and Ahmed.[6] In their review, the investigators found 12 reports, in addition to the trial by Werth and colleagues[4] discussed earlier, describing an additional 26 patients who received dapsone for treatment of their PV.[6] In these additional cases, at dosages varying between 50 and 200 mg/d, 24 of the 26 (92%) patients responded to dapsone alone or in addition to other systemic immunomodulators. In 16 of these reported cases, dapsone was added to prednisone presumably as a steroid-sparing agent, although this was not explicitly stated in every study. In 10 of these 16 patients (63%), prednisone doses were reduced after initiation of dapsone. In 6 of 16 patients (38%), prednisone dosages could not be decreased because of either continued disease or adverse events associated with dapsone. Overall, dapsone was discontinued because of adverse effects in only 4 of the 26 (15%) patients, 3 secondary to hemolysis and 1 secondary to dapsone syndrome.[6]

PF causes disease similar to PV, with the key clinical difference being that mucosal surfaces are spared in PF. Of the 10 published reports summarized by Gürcan and colleagues,[6] 9 are reports of dapsone use in only a single patient. Basset and colleagues[7] reported 9 additional patients with PF treated with dapsone in a case series published in 1987. Of the total 18 patients reported in the literature, 14 (78%) responded to dapsone at doses of 25 to 300 mg/d alone or in combination with systemic prednisone.[6] Of the 18 patients, 6 had adverse events (33%) and 2 (11%) required discontinuation of dapsone therapy (one patient because of peripheral neuropathy and the other because of dapsone-induced hypersensitivity).[6]

PEMPHIGOID

Bullous pemphigoid (BP) affects both mucosal and cutaneous surfaces. In contrast to PV, BP may remit spontaneously and can often be treated with lower doses of immunosuppressives.[2] A Cochrane review published in 2010 did not identify any randomized controlled trials evaluating dapsone as a therapy for BP.[8] The 2009 review by Gürcan and Ahmed[6] summarized the available case series and concluded that there are at least 6 published studies encompassing 170 patients with BP who received dapsone. Of these patients, 139 (81%) showed clinical improvement with 50 to 300 mg/d of dapsone alone or in combination with immunosuppressives. Adverse effects developed in 63 patients (37%), and 9 (5%) required discontinuation of the drug.[6]

Mucous membrane pemphigoid (MMP) differs from BP in that it is limited to mucosal surfaces. A randomized, double-blind, non–placebo-controlled trial published in 1986 compared 40 patients with ocular MMP treated for 6 months with either dapsone (2 mg/kg/d) or cyclophosphamide (2 mg/kg/d).[9,10] Cyclophosphamide was found to be superior to dapsone in this group of patients because all 20 patients (100%) treated with cyclophosphamide responded to the drug compared with 14 of 20 (70%) in the dapsone group.[9,10] The remaining data investigating dapsone for MMP are from non-randomized studies and reports. In the Gürcan review, 6 additional publications encompassing 182 patients with MMP treated with dapsone are discussed.[6] Of the 182 patients, 156 (86%) showed improvement with dapsone therapy. Twenty patients (11%) developed adverse effects that required discontinuation of dapsone.[6]

BULLOUS LUPUS ERYTHEMATOSUS

Bullous lupus erythematosus is a subtype of acute cutaneous lupus erythematosus (ACLE) characterized by subepidermal vesiculobullous skin lesions. Dapsone is occasionally used as an adjunctive treatment of cutaneous lupus erythematosus and is thought to be particularly useful in patients with bullous disease.[11] However, there is a dearth of studies in the literature evaluating its use, and published data are largely anecdotal. There are at least 19 patients with bullous ACLE reported in 12 case reports and series, and 17 (89%) showed improvement in their bullous lesions within days to weeks of initiation of 50 to 100 mg/d of dapsone therapy.[12–23] One of the 2 patients reported as a nonresponder had progression of disease after a week of dapsone 50 mg/d, but developed abnormal liver enzymes when the dose was increased to 100 mg/d requiring discontinuation of therapy.[18] Thus, it is difficult to determine whether dapsone may have been effective in this patient at a higher dose. Of the 17 patients reported as improving with dapsone, at least 8 (42%) had failed systemic glucocorticoid therapy, which prompted the addition of dapsone.[12,15,16,21,23]

EPIDERMOLYSIS BULLOSA ACQUISTA

Epidermolysis bullosa acquista (EBA) is an autoimmune blistering disease characterized by IgG autoantibodies that target type VII collagen. It is a rare disease without sex or racial predilection and has a prevalence of approximately 0.2 per million people.[24] EBA is a notoriously difficult disease to treat and typically requires therapy with glucocorticoids and additional immunosuppressives such as methotrexate, mycophenolate, or azathioprine.[24] Dapsone is occasionally used as an adjunctive treatment; although similar to bullous ACLE, published reports regarding dapsone's effectiveness in adults are sparse.[10] Hughes and Callen[25] reported a patient who responded to dapsone 150 mg/d, after failing treatment with niacinamide, tetracycline, and systemic prednisone. Two single-patient case reports note improvement with the use of dapsone in combination with systemic steroids.[26,27] A report published from Vienna in 1988 noted improvement with dapsone and corticosteroids in 2 of 3 patients,[28] and a German study from 1994 reported a patient successfully treated with colchicine after failing to respond to dapsone.[29] Cunningham and colleagues[30] reported on a patient partially treated with colchicine who showed complete improvement after the addition of dapsone 50 mg/d. Overall, 6 of the 8 (75%) reported patients with EBA treated with dapsone responded to the medication.

DERMATITIS HERPETIFORMIS

Dermatitis herpetiformis (DH) is an inflammatory skin condition associated with celiac disease. It is primarily a disease of white skin, with a multifactorial cause involving both genetics and environmental triggers.[31] Because of the association with celiac disease, the definitive treatment of DH is a gluten-free diet,[32] with pharmacologic therapy used as an adjunct until the diet becomes effective. Dapsone has long been used as the first-line therapy in this capacity.[31,33,34] Like most of the blistering diseases discussed in this review, randomized controlled trials evaluating the efficacy of dapsone in DH are lacking, and currently published data are limited to small case series.[33–35] Nonetheless, there is strong expert consensus that dapsone is highly efficacious for the treatment of DH, and it remains the only medication approved by the US Food and Drug Administration for use in this disease.[31,36]

LINEAR IgA BULLOUS DERMATOSIS

Linear IgA bullous dermatosis (LABD) is an immunobullous disease that has been recognized as a unique entity since the 1980s.[37] Classically, LABD has features similar to BP and DH and can be distinguished by linear IgA deposition on direct immunofluorescence. Dapsone is regarded as the first-line therapy for LABD, but, as with DH, the evidence in adults is largely based on small case reports, case series, and anecdotal evidence.[37–41] Treatment is generally started at low doses and is slowly titrated to a maintenance dose of 100 to 200 mg/d in adults.[37,41]

SUMMARY

Although dapsone is regularly used in the treatment of the AIBD, large studies evaluating its effectiveness and safety are lacking. Smaller studies and isolated reports do indicate that dapsone is effective, but, to truly determine the benefits and risks of using this medication, larger studies are needed. The best data available seem to be in MMP and PV because evidence from randomized controlled trials has been published. In addition, there seems to be wide consensus that dapsone should be the first-line pharmacologic therapy for DH and LABD. When used, the lowest effective dose should be prescribed up to a maximum of 200 mg/d, although doses up to 300 mg/d have been reported.[6] Before initiation of dapsone therapy, patients should be screened for glucose-6-phosphate dehydrogenase deficiency because patients with decreased activity of this enzyme show an approximately 2-fold increased sensitivity toward development of hemolysis.[1] In addition, a complete blood cell count with reticulocyte count should be checked weekly during the initial titration of dapsone dose, then every 2 weeks for the first 3 months, and then every 3 months after that for the development of hemolytic anemia and agranulocytosis. Liver enzymes, electrolytes, and urinalysis should also be monitored when using dapsone. Peripheral neuropathy, although rare, is a well-described adverse effect of dapsone, and periodic screening for both motor and sensory neuropathy is warranted.[1]

REFERENCES

1. Zhu YI, Stiller MJ. Dapsone and sulfones in dermatology: overview and update. J Am Acad Dermatol 2001;45(3):420–34.
2. Mutasim DF. Therapy of autoimmune bullous diseases. Ther Clin Risk Manag 2007;3(1):29–40.
3. Winkelmann RK, Roth HL. Dermatitis herpetiformis with acantholysis or pemphigus with response to sulfonamides: report of two cases. Arch Dermatol 1960;82: 385–90.
4. Werth VP, Fivenson D, Pandya AG, et al. Multicenter randomized, double-blind, placebo-controlled, clinical trial of dapsone as a glucocorticoid-sparing agent in maintenance-phase pemphigus vulgaris. Arch Dermatol 2008;144(1):25–32.

5. Martin LK, Werth V, Villanueva E, et al. Interventions for pemphigus vulgaris and pemphigus foliaceus. Cochrane Database Syst Rev 2009;1:CD006263.
6. Gürcan HM, Ahmed AR. Efficacy of dapsone in the treatment of pemphigus and pemphigoid: analysis of current data. Am J Clin Dermatol 2009;10(6):383–96.
7. Basset N, Guillot B, Michel B, et al. Dapsone as initial treatment in superficial pemphigus. Report of nine cases. Arch Dermatol 1987;123(6):783–5.
8. Kirtschig G, Middleton P, Bennett C, et al. Interventions for bullous pemphigoid. Cochrane Database Syst Rev 2010;10:CD002292.
9. Foster CS. Cicatricial pemphigoid. Trans Am Ophthalmol Soc 1986;84:527–663.
10. Kirtschig G, Murrell D, Wojnarowska F, et al. Interventions for mucous membrane pemphigoid/cicatricial pemphigoid and epidermolysis bullosa acquisita: a systematic literature review. Arch Dermatol 2002;138(3):380–4.
11. Walling HW, Sontheimer RD. Cutaneous lupus erythematosus: issues in diagnosis and treatment. Am J Clin Dermatol 2009;10(6):365–81.
12. Aboobaker J, Ramsaroop R, Abramowitz I, et al. Bullous systemic erythematosus. A case report. S Afr Med J 1986;69(1):49–51.
13. Alarcon GS, Sams WM Jr, Barton DD, et al. Bullous lupus erythematosus rash worsened by dapsone. Arthritis Rheum 1984;27(9):1071–2.
14. Burrows NP, Bhogal BS, Black MM, et al. Bullous eruption of systemic lupus erythematosus: a clinicopathological study of four cases. Br J Dermatol 1993; 128(3):332–8.
15. Fujimoto W, Hamada T, Yamada J, et al. Bullous systemic lupus erythematosus as an initial manifestation of SLE. J Dermatol 2005;32(12):1021–7.
16. Hall RP, Lawley TJ, Smith HR, et al. Bullous eruption of systemic lupus erythematosus. Dramatic response to dapsone therapy. Ann Intern Med 1982;97(2):165–70.
17. Ludgate MW, Greig DE. Bullous systemic lupus erythematosus responding to dapsone. Australas J Dermatol 2008;49(2):91–3.
18. Prystowsky JH, Finkel L, Tar L, et al. Bullous eruption in a woman with lupus erythematosus. Bullous systemic lupus erythematosus (SLE). Arch Dermatol 1988;124(4):571, 574–5.
19. Shirahama S, Yagi H, Furukawa F, et al. A case of bullous systemic lupus erythematosus. Dermatology 1994;189(Suppl 1):95–6.
20. Sirka CS, Padhi T, Mohanty P, et al. Bullous systemic lupus erythematosus: response to dapsone in two patients. Indian J Dermatol Venereol Leprol 2005; 71(1):54–6.
21. Tani M, Shimizu R, Ban M, et al. Systemic lupus erythematosus with vesiculobullous lesions. Immunoelectron microscopic studies. Arch Dermatol 1984;120(11): 1497–501.
22. Tay YK, Wong SN, Tan T. Bullous systemic lupus erythematosus—a case report and review. Ann Acad Med Singapore 1995;24(6):879–82.
23. Yung A, Oakley A. Bullous systemic lupus erythematosus. Australas J Dermatol 2000;41(4):234–7.
24. Ishii N, Hamada T, Dainichi T, et al. Epidermolysis bullosa acquisita: what's new? J Dermatol 2010;37(3):220–30.
25. Hughes AP, Callen JP. Epidermolysis bullosa acquisita responsive to dapsone therapy. J Cutan Med Surg 2001;5(5):397–9.
26. Luke MC, Darling TN, Hsu R, et al. Mucosal morbidity in patients with epidermolysis bullosa acquisita. Arch Dermatol 1999;135(8):954–9.
27. Taniuchi K, Inaoki M, Nishimura Y, et al. Nonscarring inflammatory epidermolysis bullosa acquisita with esophageal involvement and linear IgG deposits. J Am Acad Dermatol 1997;36(2 Pt 2):320–2.

28. Rappersberger K, Konrad K, Schenk P, et al. Acquired epidermolysis bullosa. A clinico-pathologic study. Hautarzt 1988;39(6):355–62 [in German].

29. Megahed M, Scharffetter-Kochanek K. Epidermolysis bullosa acquisita—successful treatment with colchicine. Arch Dermatol Res 1994;286(1):35–46.

30. Cunningham BB, Kirchmann TT, Woodley D. Colchicine for epidermolysis bullosa acquisita. J Am Acad Dermatol 1996;34(5 Pt 1):781–4.

31. Caproni M, Antiga E, Melani L, et al. Guidelines for the diagnosis and treatment of dermatitis herpetiformis. J Eur Acad Dermatol Venereol 2009;23(6):633–8.

32. Garioch JJ, Lewis HM, Sargent SA, et al. 25 years' experience of a gluten-free diet in the treatment of dermatitis herpetiformis. Br J Dermatol 1994;131(4):541–5.

33. Alexander JO. Dapsone in the treatment of dermatitis herpetiformis. Lancet 1955; 268(6876):1201–2.

34. Morgan JK, Marsden CW, Coburn JG, et al. Dapsone in dermatitis herpetiformis. Lancet 1955;268(6876):1197–200.

35. DeMento FJ, Grover RW. Acantholytic herpetiform dermatitis. Arch Dermatol 1973;107(6):883–7.

36. Junkins-Hopkins JM. Dermatitis herpetiformis: pearls and pitfalls in diagnosis and management. J Am Acad Dermatol 2010;63(3):526–8.

37. Egan CA, Zone JJ. Linear IgA bullous dermatosis. Int J Dermatol 1999;38(11): 818–27.

38. Provost TT, Maize JC, Ahmed AR, et al. Unusual subepidermal bullous diseases with immunologic features of bullous pemphigoid. Arch Dermatol 1979;115(2): 156–60.

39. Wojnarowska F. Linear IgA dapsone responsive bullous dermatosis. J R Soc Med 1980;73(5):371–3.

40. Long SA, Argenyi ZB, Piette WW. Arciform blistering in an elderly woman. Linear IgA dermatosis (LAD). Arch Dermatol 1988;124(11):1705, 1708.

41. Patricio P, Ferreira C, Gomes MM, et al. Autoimmune bullous dermatoses: a review. Ann N Y Acad Sci 2009;1173:203–10.

The Use of Intravenous Immunoglobulin in Autoimmune Bullous Diseases

Shien-Ning Chee, MBBS (UNSW)[a,b],
Dédée F. Murrell, MA, BMBCh, FAAD, MD, FACD[c,*]

KEYWORDS

- Intravenous immunoglobulin • Pemphigus
- Autoimmune bullous disease • Inflammatory disease

Autoimmune blistering diseases (AIBD) are a rare group of diseases that affects the skin and mucous membranes. They tend to be chronic remitting conditions, which have implications on best treatment and quality of life. AIBD includes pemphigus and its subtypes: bullous pemphigoid (BP), linear IgA bullous dermatosis, mucous membrane pemphigoid (MMP), and epidermolysis bullosa acquisita (EBA). There are two major categories dependent of whether the blistering is intraepidermal (pemphigus) or subepidermal (BP).

The mainstay of treatment of AIBD is corticosteroids, with doses and route of administration dependant on the type of AIBD. With exacerbations and relapses of blistering, the dose of prednisone is increased and, later, slowly tapered according to clinical response. Other immunosuppressive agents are used for a steroid-sparing effect because corticosteroids cause a significant number of side effects, including immune suppression, diabetes mellitus, osteoporosis, myopathy, cataracts, hypertension, mood changes, and peptic ulcer disease, all of which add to disease burden. Immunosuppressive agents often used include azathioprine and mycophenolate. However, these in turn have their own side effects, including bone marrow suppression, which may lead to anemia, leucopenia and thrombocytopenia, and liver

A version of this article was previously published in *Dermatologic Clinics 29:4.*

[a] Department of Dermatology, St George Hospital, Gray Street, Kogarah, Sydney, NSW 2217, Australia; [b] Faculty of Medicine, University of New South Wales, High Street, Kensington, Sydney, NSW 2052, Australia; [c] Department of Dermatology, St George Hospital, University of New South Wales, Gray Street, Kogarah, Sydney, NSW 2217, Australia
* Corresponding author.
E-mail address: d.murrell@unsw.edu.au

function abnormalities. Intravenous immunoglobulin (IVIG) is a third-line adjunctive approach to treat AIBD unresponsive to conventional therapy.[1]

INTRODUCTION TO IVIG

IVIG is made of IgG fractionated from pooled plasma, via whole blood donors or by plasmapheresis. Since its introduction in the 1950s in subcutaneous or intramuscular form, and its availability in intravenous (IV) form in the 1980s, administration has increased dramatically for a wide variety of diseases. It is used mainly in two situations. First, as replacement therapy in patients with antibody deficiency diseases— these are usually genetic conditions that have onset in early childhood. The second use is in autoimmune or inflammatory diseases.[2]

Each plasma pool of IVIG ranges from 4000 to 50,000 L, preferably from more than 1000 donors per lot. IVIG lots are not identical, with each containing varying amounts of IgG subclasses and other proteins and immunoglobulins such as albumin, IgA, IgE, and IgM.[3] Each step in production (fractionation, purification, stabilization, viral inactivation, formulation) and the varying plasma sources can exert an influence on the final product, including an effect on the biologic activity of the IgG molecule.[3]

The majority of side effects, including headache, nausea, fever, and cough, are transient and do not require discontinuation of therapy. Most of these are preventable by the administration of oral antihistamines before the infusion or slowing of the infusion rate. However, rare and potentially fatal adverse events include anaphylactic reactions, aseptic meningitis, acute renal failure, cardiovascular compromise from fluid overload, and thromboembolic events such as cerebral infraction and pulmonary emboli. Adverse effects may be related to factors such as concentration of the IVIG (thus affected volume load) and osmolality (mostly due to sodium and sugar content, possibly affecting thromboembolic events).[3,4] There are also social problems related to the use of IVIG. It is a very expensive drug, with laboratory tests, infusion equipment, and facility fees adding to the cost. It is also time consuming, with patients having to travel and take time from their normal activities for infusions.[5] The concentration of IVIG is usually 5% to 6%.[6] A higher concentration allows for smaller volumes, which is useful in patients who have conditions such as heart failure where fluid balance is a concern. Most are delivered by IV infusions, but it may also be given subcutaneously. Subcutaneous administration is helpful in patients who experience severe rate-related adverse reactions, have poor venous access, or want the convenience of self-administration. The monthly IV dose is converted into grams, then milliliters, for weekly subcutaneous administration. A subcutaneous dose of 137% of the IV dose may be needed to achieve a comparable metabolic rate. Adults usually tolerate 15 to 20 mL per infusion site.[7]

Pemphigus

Pemphigus is characterized by loss of adhesion between keratinocytes, giving rise to blister formation. This loss of adhesion is due to auto-antibodies directed against intercellular adhesion structures (acantholysis). The subtypes of pemphigus may be distinguished by the specificity of the auto-antibodies for different targets or by the location of blister formation. In the most common form, pemphigus vulgaris (PV), blisters are located just above the basal skin layer. The hallmark is flaccid blisters that easily rupture to leave denuded painful erosions, often with oral involvement. With pemphigus foliaceus (PF), blisters occur within the granular layer of the epidermis. There are superficial blisters that easily rupture to leave superficial erosions. Cutaneous involvement is often more extensive than in PV, but mucous membrane involvement is uncommon. Other pemphigus variants include paraneoplastic and drug-induced pemphigus. The titer of autoantibodies detected by indirect immunofluorescence microscopy and ELISA against desmogleins 1 and 3 in pemphigus is related to disease activity.[1,8]

IVIG is believed to work by rapidly and selectively lowering serum levels of these pathogenic antibodies that mediate pemphigus. This may be achieved by increasing catabolism of the immunoglobulin molecules. Cytotoxic agents given in conjunction with IVIG may reduce the rebound increase in levels of the depleted antibody after administration of IVIG.[9] Typically, pemphigus patients commenced on IVIG as a third-line treatment are given IVIG in addition to their oral corticosteroid and oral adjunctive agent, to which they were not responding adequately.

There have been numerous small studies, investigating the use of IVIG in PV and PF. In general, these studies show that IVIG is effective, even more so when administered concurrently with a cytotoxic drug such as cyclophosphamide or azathioprine. The addition of a cytotoxic drug is thought to offset the rebound in the level of antibodies that occurs after IVIG treatment.[9–11] However, these studies were not all placebo-controlled, randomized, or double-blinded.

The first placebo-controlled study investigating the use of IVIG in PV involved a single patient who had multiple relapses of PV despite treatment with steroids and adjunctive immunosuppressants. The patient was never disease-free and had many complications related to steroid use, including diabetes, osteopenia, ruptured tendons, and cutaneous infections secondary to immunosuppression. In 2004, all adjuvant therapies except azathioprine were discontinued, and he was placed on 140 g (2 g/kg) IVIG fortnightly for eight infusions, which led to dramatic improvement and allowed for a reduction in prednisolone from 45 to 30 mg daily. He was maintained on 80 g (1 g/kg) of IVIG monthly for 16 months. Thereafter, a formal randomized, double-blind, placebo-controlled, crossover trial was commenced. There were two phases of the trial, each consisting of 6 consecutive months of either IVIG 1 g/kg or placebo infusion. Prednisolone was continued during the trial with instructions given to the patient to taper the dose by 5 mg decrements at fortnightly intervals when lesions became quiescent and azathioprine was continued throughout at an unchanged dose. The mean subjective patient disease scores were much improved with IVIG compared with placebo (mean overall score of 11.6 vs 20.6). Also improved were pemphigus autoantibody titers (1:20 on placebo vs 1:80 with IVIG), desmoglein 3 antibody levels (79 vs 126), and desmoglein 1 antibody levels (94 vs 126). On placebo, the mean dose of prednisolone was 33.7 compared with 35.8 mg on IVIG, which is of questionable significance because there was no attempt in the protocol to taper the steroid using a standard method during the 6-month periods.[10]

There has been only one multicenter, randomized, placebo-controlled, double-blinded trial conducted in pemphigus vulgaris that were unresponsive to standard treatments or relapsing. This study was based in Japan, using patients who were unresponsive to prednisone doses over 20 mg/day. It investigated the effect of a single 5-day cycle of IVIG. Twenty-one patients were given 400 mg IVIG daily (2 g over 5 days; for a 70 kg patient equivalent to 2.5 mg/kg), 20 were given 200 mg IVIG daily, and 20 were given a placebo identical solution. There was a significant difference between the 400 mg and placebo groups in terms of therapeutic endpoint, defined as time to escape from the protocol (a novel efficacy indicator). There was also improvement with 200 mg versus placebo, but this did not reach statistical significance. Clinical severity improved significantly with both 400 mg and 200 mg compared with placebo, though the 200 mg group needed an additional 42 days to reach the same level of improvement as the 400 mg group. Antidesmoglein 3 IgG autoantibodies decreased significantly with 400 mg, decreased slightly with 200 mg, and not at all with placebo. Unlike most previous studies that suggest efficacy of IVIG for treatment of pemphigus with multiple treatment cycles, Amagai and colleagues[12] (2009) show that a single 5-day cycle has therapeutic benefits.

BP

IVIG has been reported only in uncontrolled studies of BP and found to be somewhat effective. One study investigated 15 patients who had with relapsing BP despite treatment with prednisone or systemic therapies. Data was collated regarding prednisone regimes, side effects from treatment, hospital admissions, disease activity, and quality of life as measured on a five-point Likert scale. IVIG was then initiated at 2 g/kg over 3 days every 4 weeks and prednisone and adjuvant treatments were tapered. However, patients had twice daily baths or normal saline compresses to remove skin debris followed by medium-strength topical corticosteroid cream applied to improve healing and any lesions unresponsive to topical therapy were treated with sublesional injections of 15 to 20 mg/ml of triamcinolone acetonide. This practice could have compounded the assessment of the IVIG, because topical steroids have since been shown to be effective for BP. Hence, the conclusions on demonstration of efficacy are limited from this study.[13]

Another study, coordinated by Ahmed and colleagues (2003),[14] involved 10 patients with severe BP. Serum samples were collected monthly over the study duration of 18 months to measure autoantibody titers. IVIG was administered at 4-week intervals at 2 g/kg per cycle until all lesions had healed. Thereafter the intervals between cycles were gradually increased to 6, 8, 10, 12, and 16 weeks. The mean autoantibody titers before IVIG were 2600 for BP Ag1 and 2380 for BP Ag2. After 3 months of treatment, there was clinical improvement with a statistically significant decrease in mean autoantibody titers. After 11 months, autoantibody tires became nondetectable and lesions had completely healed with no new lesions. Serologic remission was sustained for an average of 7 months with no new blister formation seen for the remainder of the study. Antibody titers to tetanus toxoid were used as controls and no change in tetanus toxoid levels was observed during the study. There was also a control group consisting of seven patients with BP in remission, seven patients with PV, and 15 healthy individuals. Antibody titers to BP Ag1 and Ag2 were nondetectable in the control group. This was the first study demonstrating the serologic response of two autoantibodies to BP when IVIG is administered. It is unknown if the patients were taking steroids or immunosuppressants before or during the study, or if their disease had been refractory to other treatments.[14] The two above studies also originate from the same study center and patient registry numbers are unavailable for tracking.

Bystryn and colleagues (2008)[15] suggest IVIG to be effective only when administered with an immunosuppressive agent. One patient with BP refractory to prednisone and mycophenolate mofetil was commenced on three cycles of IVIG given 3 weeks apart. Serum IgG decreased from 320 to 20, serum IgG4 decreased from 640 to 80 existing lesions completely cleared, and no new lesions developed. Several months later mycophenolate mofetil had been ceased and prednisone tapered to 5 mg/daily. Three cycles of IVIG every 2 weeks was administered with prednisone alone, with no improvement. In fact, serum titers of pemphigoid IgG remained unchanged, levels of IgG4 doubled, and the patient experienced one flare of disease with several new bullae. Azathioprine 150 to 200 mg/day was then added and, after four cycles of IVIG every 2 weeks, serum IgG and IgG4 halved. With another 6 cycles of IVIG, autoantibody levels decreased fourfold. However, disease activity did not correlate because there were several new bullae. Azathioprine was then ceased and IVIG was given with prednisone alone. IgG and IgG4 titers quadrupled over 3 months with an average of one new blister per week. Administration of an immunosuppressive agent with IVIG and prednisone appears to be more effective than IVIG and prednisone alone.[15]

IVIG may also be useful as monotherapy in childhood BP. A 3-month-old boy with BP was unresponsive to prednisone (2.8 mg/kg/day), dexamethasone, erythromycin, and dapsone, with new blisters and erythema over the whole body. After 2 months in hospital trialing the above treatments, a 5-day course of IVIG (300 mg/kg/day) was commenced in addition to dexamethasone 0/75 mg/day, erythromycin, and dapsone. After 4 days, no new skins lesions developed. One week later, skin lesions were much improved allowing for tapering of dexamethasone and discontinuation of erythromycin. A month later there was recurrence of blistering and a second course of IVIG was given, resulting in improvement, which allowed for discontinuation of dapsone and complete tapering of dexamethasone 7 months later. At follow-up 16 months later, there had been no relapse.[16] Another case involved a Chinese, 3-month-old boy with BP and eczema, whose parents refused systemic steroid therapy. IVIG 400 mg/kg/day was given for 4 days with cefaclor. Erythema and most bullae over the body resolved within 1 week. Within the next year, there were several mild relapses of blisters that were controlled with oral antihistamines and topical corticosteroids. In the following 2 years, there were no relapses of bullae.[17]

MMP

MMP affects the mucous membranes of the body, including the oral cavity, ocular membranes, nose, pharynx, larynx, trachea, and genitalia. Ocular involvement can ultimately lead to blindness.[18]

There has been one comparison study involving 18 patients with ocular MMP. Eight patients were treated with IVIG, and then compared with eight other patients on conventional immunosuppressive therapy who had identical disease (duration and severity) and were matched for age and sex. The IVIG group was given 2 g/kg per cycle of 2 to 4 week intervals. Once clinical improvement was observed and disease had stabilized, the previous systemic conventional therapy was discontinued, but the method for tapering was not specified. IVIG continued for 16 weeks. Conventional therapy differed between patients, including agents such as prednisone, diaminodiphenylsulfone (dapsone), methotrexate, azathioprine, or mycophenolate mofetil. All patients in the IVIG group had total control of disease at 24 months with no progression of disease, while the other group had disease progression despite using conventional therapy at adequate doses for recommended periods of time. IVIG users also had faster control of ocular inflammation and no relapses, unlike patients on conventional therapy. Letko and colleagues[19] (2004) suggest that ocular MMP should be an indication for IVIG treatment.

Another pilot study of six patients with severe ocular involvement unresponsive to conventional therapy also demonstrated the efficacy of IVIG (cycles of 2 g/kg over 3 days), with rapid improvement in symptoms and signs such as conjunctival erythema, photophobia, and discomfort. No patients had a decrease in their disease staging and two patients had an improvement. This study is continuing, investigating the durability of long-term remission.[20]

Three other case studies have found IVIG to be effective in recalcitrant MMP. In these studies, IVIG was given in addition to steroids with or without immunosuppressants. Two studies used IVIG 1 g/kg/daily for 2 to 3 days. One study did not quantify the amount of IVIG given.[21–23]

EBA

EBA is characterized by inflammatory or noninflammatory blisters at sites of trauma that affect the collagen VII under the lamina densa, thus leading to milia and scar formation. There are various types of EBA, some of which resemble BP or MMP.[1] There have been few case studies on the use of IVIG in EBA.

One study involving a 16-year-old boy showed that high-dose IVIG (400 mg/kg/day for 4 days repeated every 2 weeks) led to good clinical improvement when administered with cyclosporin and prednisone. However, there was no decrease in circulating autoantibodies.[24] There have been two studies investigating high-dose IVIG without concomitant use of steroids or immunosuppressants. One of these studies showed improvement after two cycles of IVIG (400 mg/kg/day for 5 days) with healing of most erosions and few new blisters. Six months after the sixth and final cycle, the condition was still in remission.[25] However, the other study showed no improvement in disease either clinically or by measurement of autoantibodies.[26]

Low-dose IVIG is an alternative that allows for reduced costs and side effects. One patient with EBA refractory to steroids, immunosuppressants, colchicine, and plasmapheresis was commenced on IVIG at 40 mg/daily in 3-day cycles repeated every 3 to 4 weeks, coadministered with prednisone. After four cycles, no new blisters appeared and lesions started healing. One year later, prednisone was discontinued and the interval between IVIG infusions was extended to 6 weeks. To the time of publication of the case-study, the patient remained disease-free and continued to receive low-dose IVIG every 6 weeks.[27]

IVIG has also successfully been administered subcutaneously. One patient with EBA resistant to corticosteroids, azathioprine, mycophenolate mofetil, mercaptopurine, minocycline, and plasmapheresis was given two boluses of 1.7 g/kg IVIG at 8 weekly intervals, followed by divided doses every 3 weeks. Treatment was changed to subcutaneous immunoglobulin (SCIG) due to poor venous access and convenience of self-treatment at home. Throughout treatment with both IVIG and SCIG, there was reduction of symptoms and gradual withdrawal of all immunosuppressive therapy. Maintenance was achieved with SCIG at 0.9 g/kg/month given in divided doses on 5 days per week. Circulating autoantibodies reduced from 1:16 to zero on intact skin, and 1:32 to 1:10 on salt split skin testing. Subcutaneous administration may be a good alternative in patients with poor venous access, or those who wish to be able to administer their medication at home.[28]

SUMMARY

IVIG has been shown to be effective in the treatment of AIBD and may be an option if disease is refractory to conventional treatment. Effectiveness of IVIG appears to increase when administered concurrently with a cytotoxic drug. Most reports use multiple treatment cycles, though single cycles may give benefit. Tapering IVIG administration may improve the duration of remission and subcutaneous injections may be an option if IVIG is inconvenient or inappropriate.

There is a need for well-conducted, randomized, placebo-controlled double-blinded trials investigating the use of IVIG in AIBD, particularly in BP, MMP, and EBA, so that patients can receive good, evidence-based care. Issues requiring more investigation include

Optimal IVIG doses and regimens (eg, number of cycles, intervals between cycles, use of tapering of IVIG, when IVIG should be first commenced)
Benefits of adjuvant immunosuppressive agents
Relative benefits of agents

Cost-effectiveness
Effectiveness of IVIG in modification or suppression of the course of disease.

REFERENCES

1. Ahmed A. Use of intravenous immunoglobulin therapy in autoimmune blistering diseases. Int Immunopharmacol 2006;6:557–78.
2. Gelfand E. Differences between IGIV products: impact on clinical outcome. Int Immunopharmacol 2006;6:592–9.
3. Martin T. IGIV: contents, properties, and methods of industrial production—evolving closer to a more physiologic product. Int Immunopharmacol 2006;6: 517–22.
4. Feldmeyer L, Benden C, Haile S, et al. Not all intravenous immunoglobulin preparations are equally well tolerated. Acta Derm Venereol 2010;90(5):494–7.
5. Dahl M, Bridges A. Intravenous immune globulin: fighting antibodies with antibodies. J Am Acad Dermatol 2001;45(5):775–84.
6. Red Cross Australia. Appendix 1 - Comparison of INTRAGAM P, Flebogamma 5% DIF and Octagam. 2011. Available at: http://www.transfusion.com.au/sites/default/files/Comparison%20between%20IVIG%20products%20-%20Final.pdf. Accessed June 24, 2011.
7. Ballow M. Immunoglobulin therapy: methods of delivery. J Allergy Clin Immunol 2008;122(5):1038–9.
8. Nousari H, Anhalt G. Pemphigus and bullous pemphigoid. Lancet 1999;354: 667–72.
9. Lolis M, Toosi S, Czernick A, et al. Effect of intravenous immunoglobulin with or without cytotoxic drugs on pemphigus intercellular antibodies. J Am Acad Dermatol 2011;64(3):484–9.
10. Arnold D, Burton J, Shine B, et al. An 'n-of-1' placebo-controlled crossover trial of intravenous immunoglobulin as adjuvant therapy in refractory pemphigus vulgaris. Br J Dermatol 2009;160(5):1098–102.
11. Bystryn J, Jiao D, Natow S. Treatment of pemphigus with intravenous immunoglobulin. J Am Acad Dermatol 2002;47(3):358–63.
12. Amagai M, Ikeda S, Shimizu H, et al. A randomised double-blind trial of intravenous immunoglobulin for pemphigus. J Am Acad Dermatol 2009;60(4):595–603.
13. Ahmed A. Intravenous immunoglobulin therapy for patients with bullous pemphigoid unresponsive to conventional immunosuppressive treatment. J Am Acad Dermatol 2001;45(6):825–35.
14. Sami N, Ali S, Bhol K, et al. Influence of intravenous immunoglobulin therapy on autoantibody titres to BP Ag1 and BP Ag2 in patients with bullous pemphigoid. J Eur Acad Dermatol Venereol 2003;17:641–5.
15. Czernik A, Bystryn J. Improvement of intravenous immunoglobulin therapy for bullous pemphigoid by adding immunosuppressive agents. Arch Dermatol 2008;144(5):658–61.
16. Sugawara N, Nagai Y, Matsushima Y, et al. Infantile bullous pemphigoid treated with intravenous immunoglobulin therapy. J Am Acad Dermatol 2007;57(6): 1084–9.
17. Xiao T, Li B, Wang Y, et al. Childhood bullous pemphigoid treated by i.v. immunoglobulin. J Dermatol 2007;34:650–3.
18. Chan L, Ahmed A, Anhalt G. The first international consensus on mucous membrane pemphigoid: definition, diagnostic criteria, pathogenic factors, medical treatment and prognostic indicators. Arch Dermatol 2002;138:370–9.

19. Letko E, Miserocchi E, Daoud Y, et al. A nonrandomized comparison of the clinical outcome of ocular involvement in patients with mucous membrane (cicatricial) pemphigoid between conventional immunosuppressive and intravenous immunoglobulin therapies. Clin Immunol 2004;111:303–10.
20. Mignogna M, Leuci S, Piscopo R, et al. Intravenous immunoglobulins and mucous membrane pemphigoid [letter]. Ophthalmology 2008;115(4):752, e751.
21. Galdos M, Etxebarria J. Intravenous immunoglobulin therapy for refractory ocular cicatricial pemphigoid: case report. Cornea 2008;27(8):967–9.
22. Leverkus M, Georgi M, Nie Z, et al. Cicatricial pemphigoid with circulating IgA and IgG autoantibodies to the central portion of the BP180 ectodomain: beneficial effect of adjuvant therapy with high-dose intravenous immunoglobulin. J Am Acad Dermatol 2002;46:116–22.
23. Iaccheri B, Roque M, Fiore T, et al. Ocular cicatricial pemphigoid, keratomycosis, and intravenous immunoglobulin therapy. Cornea 2004;23:819–22.
24. Meier F, Soninichsen K, Schaumburg-Lever G, et al. Epidermolysis bullosa acquisita: efficacy of high-dose intravenous immunoglobulins. J Am Acad Dermatol 1993;29(2):334–7.
25. Gourgiotou K, Exadaktylou D, Aroni K, et al. Epidermolysis bullosa acquisita: treatment with intravenous immunoglobulins. J Eur Acad Dermatol Venereol 2002;16:77–80.
26. Caldwell M, Yancey K, Engler R, et al. Epidermolysis bullosa acquisita: Efficacy of high-dose intravenous immunoglobulins [letter to the editor]. J Am Acad Dermatol 1994;31(5):827–8.
27. Kofler H, Wambacher-Gasser B, Topar G, et al. Intravenous immunoglobulin treatment in therapy-resistant epidermolysis bullosa acquisita. J Am Acad Dermatol 1996;36(2):331–5.
28. Tayal U, Burton J, Chapel H. Subcutaneous immunoglobulin therapy for immunomodulation in a patient with severe epidermolysis bullosa acquisita [letter to the editor]. Clin Immunol 2008;129:518–9.

Rituximab and its Use in Autoimmune Bullous Disorders

Benjamin S. Daniel, BA, BCom, MBBS, MMed (Clin Epi)[a,b],
Dédée F. Murrell, MA, BMBCh, FAAD, MD, FACD[c,*], Pascal Joly, MD, PhD[d]

KEYWORDS

• CD20 antigen • Autoimmune blistering diseases
• Immunosuppressant • Adverse effects

Rituximab is a chimeric murine-human monoclonal antibody against the CD20 antigen of B lymphocytes[1,2] (anti-CD20 mAb). It is used in multiple medical conditions and its therapeutic role in dermatology has been increasing in the last decade. Initially used in the treatment of non-Hodgkin B-cell lymphoma, the scope of rituximab has been expanded to include autoimmune diseases such as rheumatoid arthritis (RA), systemic lupus erythematosus (SLE), and chronic immune thrombocytopenic purpura syndrome.[3,4] Because the B cells produce immunoglobulins, which in turn have a pathogenic role in autoimmune diseases, their depletion is surmised to result in improved symptoms and disease control. Depleting B cells inevitably decreases the activation of antigen-presenting cells and the transmission of signaling pathways to other key mediators, such as T cells.

MECHANISM OF ACTION

The B-cell antigen CD20 is a transmembrane glycoprotein expressed on nearly all B cells and most B-cell lymphomas.[5,6] However, it is not found on early pre-B cells or stem cells.[5] B cells, originally arising from the bone marrow, mature by migrating through peripheral blood, lymph nodes, and spleen. In bone marrow (BM) they are known as plasma cells. CD20, specific for B cells, is expressed on B cells between the pre-B cell and pre-plasma stages.[7,8] Because rituximab targets CD20, plasma cells in the BM responsible for antibody production[6] are spared. Once rituximab binds

A version of this article was previously published in *Dermatologic Clinics 29:4.*
[a] Department of Dermatology, St George Hospital, Gray Street, Kogarah, Sydney, NSW 2217, Australia; [b] Faculty of Medicine, University of New South Wales, Sydney, NSW 2052, Australia; [c] Department of Dermatology, St George Hospital, University of New South Wales, Gray Street, Kogarah, Sydney, NSW 2217, Australia; [d] Dermatology Department, INSERM U905, Rouen University Hospital, 1 Rue de Germont, 76031 Rouen, France
* Corresponding author.
E-mail address: d.murrell@unsw.edu.au

Immunol Allergy Clin N Am 32 (2012) 331–337
doi:10.1016/j.iac.2012.04.013   immunology.theclinics.com
0889-8561/12/$ – see front matter © 2012 Elsevier Inc. All rights reserved.

to the CD20 protein, transmembrane signals result in altered cell-cycle differentiation and activation. Cell-mediated cytotoxicity, complement system, and direct apoptosis[9] have been implemented in the subsequent reduction in circulating CD20+ B cells in the periphery, lymph nodes, spleen, and bone marrow.[5]

The depletion of B-cell counts occurs within 3 days of rituximab administration and is reported to be reduced by about 90%, although variations occur. It is thought that the variations are due to the underlying disease and polymorphisms of FcγRIIIa receptors.[8] The B-cell count remains low for 6 months and returns to baseline around 9 to 12 months after receiving 4 weekly doses of 375 mg/m^2.[6,10] In addition to depleting B cells, some data suggest that antigen-specific CD4+ T-cell numbers are reduced after the administration of rituximab,[11] whereas no quantitative change in the different T-cell subpopulations is usually evident.[12]

DOSE AND ROUTE OF ADMINISTRATION

Although rituximab is typically prescribed in weekly infusions of 375 mg/m^2 (approx. 727.5 mg per 75 kg, 1.8 m tall male) for 4 weeks, some advocate 2 intravenous infusions of 1 g, 2 weeks apart.[4] Rituximab is also known as Rituxan or MabThera. Infusions are initially administered over 5 hours and if well tolerated, subsequent infusions can be administered over 3 to 5 hours.[10]

Corticosteroids reduce the intensity of infusion-related adverse effects.[4] Paracetamol and diphenhydramine are recommended before administration to decrease the likelihood and extent of infusion-related adverse events.[10]

Monitoring of B-cell counts does not generally affect treatment because a sharp decline in absolute numbers is expected after the administration of rituximab. The aim of recurrent cycles of rituximab is to maintain circulating B cells at the lowest level for a prolonged period of time. In one report, rituximab was administered every 6 to 9 months for RA without significant adverse effects apart from reduction in serum immunoglobulin M levels.[4] The theoretic risk of increasing the incidence of lymphomas after prolonged B-cell depletion with repeated cycles of rituximab cannot be excluded.

Routine vaccination of all patients should occur several weeks before the commencement of rituximab therapy.[4] Patients should not receive live vaccines while receiving systemic immunosuppressive agents.

ADVERSE EFFECTS

Polymorphisms of the FcγRIIIa receptor may influence the efficacy of rituximab and the extent of associated adverse effects.[9] The most frequent adverse effects are transient, infusion-related, and mild to moderate in severity.[10] They include fever, headache, nausea, chills, orthostatic hypotension, mucocutaneous reactions, and thrombocytopenia.[2,5,9] Severe cytokine release syndrome can occur during the first infusion.[10] It is of major importance not to forget infections, which can be severe. There was 1 case of septicemia leading to death in the series of 21 patients reported by Joly and colleagues,[2] 1 of 7 patients died in the series studied by Hertl,[11–13] and 2 of 17 patients died in the cicatricial pemphigoid series from St Louis,[14] which approximately corresponds to 4 deaths among 44 patients (almost 10%). These severe infections seem favored by older age and the concomitant use of high doses of steroids and/or immunosuppressants. There have been a significant number of reports of progressive multifocal leukoencephalopathy in patients concomitantly treated with rituximab and polychemotherapy for B-cell lymphoma and some reported cases in patients with nondermatologic autoimmune diseases such as SLE, RA, and Wegener granulomatosis.[9]

Although it has been theorized and confirmed by many reports that serum levels of immunoglobulin G (IgG) remain unchanged because stem cells and plasma cells do not contain CD20[15] and are not affected, few case reports have reported reduced levels of immunoglobulins.[14] Anemia, neutropenia, and thrombocytopenia have also been reported in 1% to 7% of patients after the fourth infusion.[10] In the context of these findings, it is important to regularly monitor blood counts in patients treated with rituximab.

USE IN AUTOIMMUNE BLISTERING DISEASES

Autoimmune blistering diseases (AIBD) are a heterogeneous group of blistering diseases affecting the skin and/or mucous membrane. Although these diseases are typically managed with systemic corticosteroids in combination with immunosuppressants or immunomodulators, inefficacy (recalcitrant and relapsing types), contraindications, and adverse effects are reasons for choosing an alternative therapeutic option. This is especially the case with pemphigus and mucous membrane pemphigoid, which often require prolonged administration of systemic corticosteroids and other adjuvant systemic immunosuppressive agents. Rituximab has therefore been used as an alternative and/or adjuvant to other therapies.

Pemphigus

Pemphigus is a rare mucocutaneous disease characterized by antibodies to adhesion protein, desmoglein (Dsg) 1 and 3. Pemphigus vulgaris (PV) and pemphigus foliaceus (PF) are the 2 main types of pemphigus usually managed with systemic corticosteroids. Adjuvant therapies such as mycophenolate, azathioprine, methotrexate cyclophosphamide, and cyclosporine are used with varying degrees of efficacy.[16,17]

The use of rituximab in pemphigus was first reported in 2002 and since then there have been many case reports/series demonstrating favorable results, especially in patients who have not responded to more standard treatments.[18,19] A study assessing the resolution of pemphigus lesions with intravenous immunoglobulin (IVIG) and rituximab was published in 2006.[20] Eleven patients with recalcitrant disease were treated with rituximab (375 mg/m^2) once a week for 3 weeks and with IVIG (2 g/kg) in the fourth week. This cycle was repeated for month 2. During months 3 to 6, these patients were administered one infusion of rituximab and IVIG. By the end of the second cycle, 9 of 11 patients (82%) had resolution of lesions, which was maintained for more than 20 months. The combination of IVIG with rituximab was not compared with rituximab alone, and hence it is uncertain whether IVIG adds any benefit to rituximab alone.

Two patients with recalcitrant PV were successfully treated with 2 courses of rituximab.[21] The 2 reports on these cases implied better outcomes with 2 cycles of rituximab rather than 1 but because these are only isolated case reports, it is difficult to draw any firm conclusions. In 2007, however, a multicenter open-label French trial assessing the effect of a single cycle of rituximab alone in pemphigus was reported.[2] Twenty-one patients (14 with PV, 7 with PF) who failed to respond, be maintained, or had a contraindication to oral corticosteroids were given a single cycle of rituximab. Each patient received 1 infusion (375 mg/m^2) weekly for 4 weeks, with immunologic evaluations at regular intervals. Eighteen of 21 patients (86%) had complete remission at 3 months and 2 of 21 patients (10%) had complete remission by 12 months. Of those who had complete remission, 9 (45%) patients relapsed after a mean of 19 months, 2 of whom required a second cycle of rituximab. This study also demonstrated the corticosteroid-sparing effect of rituximab, with 8 of 21 (38%) patients not requiring any systemic treatment at the end of the study. A relationship between disease activity and antidesmoglein antibody (anti-DSG) levels was evident by the reduction of anti-DSG-1 and, to a lesser degree, anti-DSG-3 titers in patients who had experienced remission at 3 months. Rituximab does not seem to influence the mean IgG levels, which did not change significantly.

In a study in 2006 from Germany, rituximab was administered to 7 patients with AIBD (4 with PV, 2 with bullous pemphigoid (BP), and 1 with mucous membrane pemphigoid [MMP]). Six of 7 patients received weekly infusions (375 mg/m^2) for 4 weeks. Although complete resolution or reduction in lesion size by more than 50% occurred in 6 of 7 patients (86%) at 13 months, 4 of 7 patients (57%) had severe adverse effects including blindness and death secondary to bacterial pneumonia.[22]

Maintenance therapy at a lower dose may be an option in the treatment of pemphigus[21] that requires further evaluation.

MMP/Epidermolysis Bullosa Acquisita

MMP refers to a heterogeneous group of AIBD typically affecting the mucous membranes.[14] MMP is associated with significant morbidity secondary to scarring and ophthalmologic complications. Typical histologic findings include IgG and C3 depositions in the basement membrane zone.[23] MMP, previously known as cicatricial pemphigoid,[24] is a potentially severe AIBD with an incidence of 1 per 1,000,000 per year with a mean age of 70 years.[25,26] Epidermolysis bullosa acquisita (EBA) has an incidence of 0.2 new cases per 1,000,000 inhabitants per year.[25,26] The use of rituximab in MMP and EBA has been limited to a few case reports.[15,27,28] Combination therapy with IVIG has been reported to be effective in ocular cicatricial pemphigoid.[20,29] In a recent study, 25 patients with severe refractory MMP were treated with 1 to 2 cycles of rituximab (375 mg/m^2) for 4 weeks.[14] Within a median of 12 weeks of having 1 cycle, 17 patients had complete resolution of their lesions. Five of the 8 remaining patients experienced complete resolution after receiving a second cycle of rituximab. Although 22 of 25 patients (88%) had complete resolution of both ocular and extraocular lesions, 10 of 22 patients (45%) had a relapse after a mean of only 4 months. Significant adverse events occurred in this study, with 3 patients experiencing infections, 2 of whom died. Despite the severity of adverse outcomes, it can be argued that in the case of MMP, it is important to quickly achieve disease stabilization and remission as disease progression often leads to blindness, laryngeal, and esophageal complications.[14] The benefits versus the risks must always be considered before administration of rituximab.

Rituximab has been suggested as a potential corticosteroid-sparing agent,[2,18] reducing cumulative doses of systemic corticosteroids, although this has not been demonstrated in a randomized controlled trial.

BP

Although BP is the most common AIBD, the use of rituximab is infrequently reported, probably because BP responds readily to potent topical corticosteroids.[30,31] Typically affecting the elderly with high mortality, BP presents with multiple bullae, erosions, and severe pruritus, and only rarely has mucous membrane involvement. Two female patients with concomitant BP and chronic lymphocytic leukemia were both treated with rituximab (375 mg/m^2 weekly for 4 consecutive weeks) alone after inadequate response to corticosteroids and antihistamines.[32] Maintenance therapy of 1 dose every 2 months was initiated and both patients had complete remission after this treatment, even at the 3-year follow-up.

Successful use of rituximab has been reported in a 5-month old infant who had unsuccessful systemic treatments including corticosteroids, dapsone, IVIG, and cyclosporine.[33] Two doses of rituximab were added to the therapeutic regimen 4 weeks apart (375 mg/m^2 and 187.5 mg/m^2), and improvement was noticed within days.

A retrospective study looking at 7 patients (5 with BP and 2 with MMP) treated with rituximab found that complete and partial remission was achieved in 4 patients with BP and 2 patients with MMP.[34] The main indications for the use of rituximab in BP patients are not clearly defined because of the extremely high efficacy of ultrapotent topical corticosteroids during the acute phase of the disease and the numerous drugs proposed for maintenance therapy (oral corticosteroids, low doses of methotrexate, tetracyclines). Potential indications for the administration of rituximab in BP might be: (1) recalcitrant types of BP (extremely rare) and (2) patients with multiple relapses, who are observed quite frequently.

SUMMARY

In recent years, many clinicians have used rituximab in an off-label way to successfully treat and manage AIBD. Although traditional systemic treatments such as corticosteroids have been effective, they are associated with multiple adverse effects and in some cases fail to adequately control symptoms. Additional therapy in the form of weekly intravenous infusions of rituximab (375 mg/m^2) may benefit patients with recalcitrant disease and allow for tapering and cessation of other systemic agents.

Rituximab induces B-cell depletion and hence a reduction in pathogenic antibodies. Long-term monitoring is advisable, given the possibility of immunocompromise and sepsis. The exact time to initiate rituximab is variable. Due to the cost, potential complications, and lack of data, it is prudent to treat AIBD with rituximab if 2 or more traditional systemic therapies have failed to adequately control symptoms.[33,34] Rituximab is a promising therapeutic agent in AIBD but further research is required.

REFERENCES

1. Carr DR, Heffernan MP. Innovative uses of rituximab in dermatology. Dermatol Clin 2010;28(3):547–57.
2. Joly P, Mouquet H, Roujeau JC, et al. A single cycle of rituximab for the treatment of severe pemphigus. N Engl J Med 2007;357(6):545–52.
3. Looney RJ. B cells as a therapeutic target in autoimmune diseases other than rheumatoid arthritis. Rheumatology (Oxford) 2005;44(Suppl 2):ii13–7.
4. Sanz I. Indications of rituximab in autoimmune diseases. Drug Discov Today Ther Strateg 2009;6(1):13–9.
5. Maloney DG, Liles TM, Czerwinski DK, et al. Phase I clinical trial using escalating single-dose infusion of chimeric anti-CD20 monoclonal antibody (IDEC-C2B8) in patients with recurrent B cell lymphoma. Blood 1994;84(8):2457–66.
6. Zambruno G, Borradori L. Rituximab immunotherapy in pemphigus: therapeutic effects beyond B cell depletion. J Invest Dermatol 2008;128(12):2745–7.
7. Edwards JC, Cambridge G. B cell targeting in rheumatoid arthritis and other autoimmune diseases. Nat Rev Immunol 2006;6(5):394–403.
8. Schmidt E, Hunzelmann N, Zillikens D, et al. Rituximab in refractory autoimmune bullous diseases. Clin Exp Dermatol 2006;31(4):503–8.
9. McDonald V, Leandro M. Rituximab in non-haematological disorders of adults and its mode of action. Br J Haematol 2009;146(3):233–46.

10. Onrust SV, Lamb HM, Balfour JA. Rituximab. Drugs 1999;58(1):79–88 [discussion: 89–90].
11. Eming R, Nagel A, Wolff-Franke S, et al. Rituximab exerts a dual effect in pemphigus vulgaris. J Invest Dermatol 2008;128(12):2850–8.
12. Mouquet H, Musette P, Gougeon ML, et al. B cell depletion immunotherapy in pemphigus: effects on cellular and humoral immune responses. J Invest Dermatol 2008;128(12):2859–69.
13. Muller R, Hunzelmann N, Baur V, et al. Targeted immunotherapy with rituximab leads to a transient alteration of the IgG autoantibody profile in pemphigus vulgaris. Dermatol Res Pract 2010;2010:321950.
14. Le Roux-Villet C, Prost-Squarcioni C, Alexandre M, et al. Rituximab for patients with refractory mucous membrane pemphigoid. Arch Dermatol 2011;147:843–9.
15. Sadler E, Schafleitner B, Lanschuetzer C, et al. Treatment-resistant classical epidermolysis bullosa acquisita responding to rituximab. Br J Dermatol 2007;157(2):417–9.
16. Daniel BS, Murrell DF. The actual management of pemphigus. G Ital Dermatol Venereol 2010;145(5):689–702.
17. Martin LK, Werth V, Villanueva E, et al. Interventions for pemphigus vulgaris and pemphigus foliaceus. Cochrane Database Syst Rev 2009;1:CD006263.
18. Fernando SL, O'Connor KS. Treatment of severe pemphigus foliaceus with rituximab. Med J Aust 2008;189(5):289–90.
19. Virgolini L, Marzocchi V. Anti-CD20 monoclonal antibody (rituximab) in the treatment of autoimmune diseases. Successful result in refractory pemphigus vulgaris: report of a case. Haematologica 2003;88(7):ELT24.
20. Ahmed AR, Spigelman Z, Cavacini LA, et al. Treatment of pemphigus vulgaris with rituximab and intravenous immune globulin. N Engl J Med 2006;355(17):1772–9.
21. Faurschou A, Gniadecki R. Two courses of rituximab (anti-CD20 monoclonal antibody) for recalcitrant pemphigus vulgaris. Int J Dermatol 2008;47(3):292–4.
22. Schmidt E, Seitz CS, Benoit S, et al. Rituximab in autoimmune bullous diseases: mixed responses and adverse effects. Br J Dermatol 2007;156(2):352–6.
23. Kirtschig G, Murrell D, Wojnarowska F, et al. Interventions for mucous membrane pemphigoid/cicatricial pemphigoid and epidermolysis bullosa acquisita: a systematic literature review. Arch Dermatol 2002;138(3):380–4.
24. Chan LS, Ahmed AR, Anhalt GJ, et al. The first international consensus on mucous membrane pemphigoid: definition, diagnostic criteria, pathogenic factors, medical treatment, and prognostic indicators. Arch Dermatol 2002;138(3):370–9.
25. Zillikens D, Wever S, Roth A, et al. Incidence of autoimmune subepidermal blistering dermatoses in a region of central Germany. Arch Dermatol 1995;131(8):957–8.
26. Bernard P, Vaillant L, Labeille B, et al. Incidence and distribution of subepidermal autoimmune bullous skin diseases in three French regions. Bullous Diseases French Study Group. Arch Dermatol 1995;131(1):48–52.
27. Niedermeier A, Eming R, Pfütze M, et al. Clinical response of severe mechanobullous epidermolysis bullosa acquisita to combined treatment with immunoadsorption and rituximab (anti-CD20 monoclonal antibodies). Arch Dermatol 2007;143(2):192–8.
28. Crichlow SM, Mortimer NJ, Harman KE. A successful therapeutic trial of rituximab in the treatment of a patient with recalcitrant, high-titer epidermolysis bullosa acquisita. Br J Dermatol 2007;156(1):194–6.

29. Foster CS, Chang PY, Ahmed AR. Combination of rituximab and intravenous immunoglobulin for recalcitrant ocular cicatricial pemphigoid: a preliminary report. Ophthalmology 2010;117(5):861–9.
30. Joly P, Roujeau JC, Benichou J, et al, Bullous Diseases French Study Group. A comparison of oral and topical corticosteroids in patients with bullous pemphigoid. N Engl J Med 2002;346(5):321–7.
31. Langan SM, Smeeth L, Hubbard R, et al. Bullous pemphigoid and pemphigus vulgaris–incidence and mortality in the UK: population based cohort study. BMJ 2008;337:a180.
32. Saouli Z, Papadopoulos A, Kaiafa G, et al. A new approach on bullous pemphigoid therapy. Ann Oncol 2008;19(4):825–6.
33. Schulze J, Bader P, Henke U, et al. Severe bullous pemphigoid in an infant–successful treatment with rituximab. Pediatr Dermatol 2008;25(4):462–5.
34. Lourari S, Herve C, Doffoel-Hantz V, et al. Bullous and mucous membrane pemphigoid show a mixed response to rituximab: experience in seven patients. J Eur Acad Dermatol Venereol 2010. [Epub ahead of print].

Index

Note: Page numbers of article titles are in **boldface** type.

A

Acantholysis, in pemphigus vulgaris, 238
Achlorhydria, in dermatitis herpetiformis, 265
Autoimmune skin diseases. *See also specific diseases and drugs.*
    azathioprine for, **295–307**
    bullous pemphigoid
        clinical features of, **217–232**
        pathogenesis of, **207–215**
    corticosteroids for, **283–294**
    dapsone for, **317–322**
    dermatitis herpetiformis. *See* Dermatitis herpetiformis.
    intravenous immunoglobulin for, **323–330**
    linear IgA disease, **245–253**
    mycophenolate mofetil for, **309–315**
    pemphigus vulgaris, **233–243**
    rituximab for, **331–337**
Azathioprine, **295–307**
    for bullous pemphigoid, 297
    for pemphigus, 297–300
    history of, 295
    in pregnancy, 299, 301
    metabolism of, 295–297
    side effects of, 301–304
    structure of, 295–296

B

Betamethasone, 285–286, 288
Biopsy
    for bullous pemphigoid, 223–224
    for pemphigus vulgaris, 237–238
Blisters
    in bullous pemphigoid, 218–226
    in dermatitis herpetiformis, 256–258, 264
    in linear IgA disease, **245–253**
    in pemphigus vulgaris, 233–238
Bone loss, from corticosteroids, 290–291
BP180 protein (collagen type XVII, COL 17, BPAG2 protein)
    in bullous pemphigoid, 207–213, 222–226
    in linear IgA disease, 250

Immunol Allergy Clin N Am 32 (2012) 339–346
doi:10.1016/S0889-8561(12)00038-0
0889-8561/12/$ – see front matter © 2012 Elsevier Inc. All rights reserved.

immunology.theclinics.com

Moving?

Make sure your subscription moves with you!

To notify us of your new address, find your **Clinics Account Number** (located on your mailing label above your name), and contact customer service at:

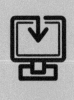

Email: **journalscustomerservice-usa@elsevier.com**

800-654-2452 (subscribers in the U.S. & Canada)
314-447-8871 (subscribers outside of the U.S. & Canada)

Fax number: 314-447-8029

Elsevier Health Sciences Division
Subscription Customer Service
3251 Riverport Lane
Maryland Heights, MO 63043

*To ensure uninterrupted delivery of your subscription, please notify us at least 4 weeks in advance of move.

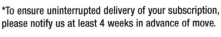

Printed and bound by CPI Group (UK) Ltd, Croydon, CR0 4YY

03/10/2024

01040439-0016